A LITTLE BOOK OF SELF CARE

AYURVEDA

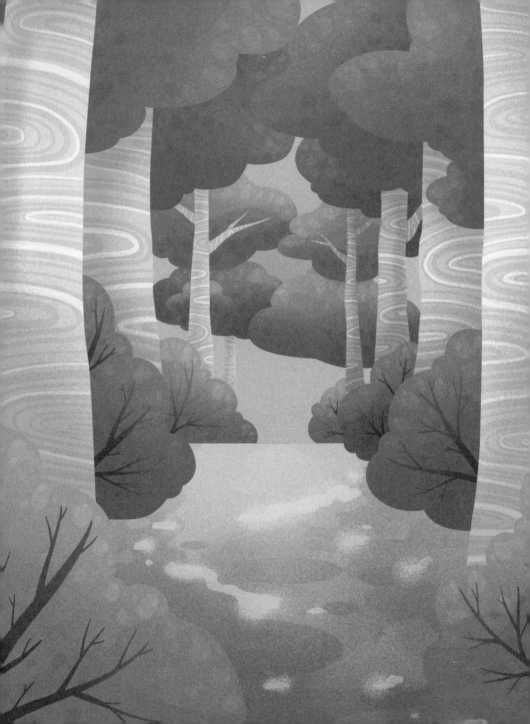

A LITTLE BOOK OF SELF CARE

AYURVEDA

AN ANCIENT SYSTEM OF HOLISTIC HEALTH TO BRING
BALANCE AND WELLNESS TO YOUR LIFE

SONJA SHAH-WILLIAMS

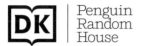

Editor Aimée Longos
Designer Mandy Earey
Senior Editor Rona Skene
Project Art Editor Louise Brigenshaw
Editorial Assistant Kiron Gill
Jacket Designer Amy Cox
Jackets Coordinator Lucy Philpott
Senior Production Editor Tony Phipps
Production Controller Rebecca Parton
Creative Technical Support
Sonia Charbonnier
Managing Editor Dawn Henderson
Managing Art Editor Marianne Markham
Art Director Maxine Pedliham
Publishing Director Mary-Clare Jerram

Illustrated by Weitong Mai

First published in Great Britain in 2020 by
Dorling Kindersley Limited
DK, One Embassy Gardens, 8 Viaduct Gardens,
London, SW11 7BW

Copyright © 2020 Dorling Kindersley Limited

A Penguin Random House Company
10 9 8 7 6 5 4 3 2 1
001–318950–Dec/2020

DISCLAIMER see page 144

A CIP catalogue record for this book
is available from the British Library.
ISBN: 978-0-2414-4365-1

Printed and bound in China

For the curious
www.dk.com

MIX
Paper from
responsible sources
FSC™ C018179

This book was made with Forest
Stewardship Council ™ certified
paper – one small step in DK's
commitment to a sustainable
future. For more information go to
www.dk.com/our-green-pledge

CONTENTS

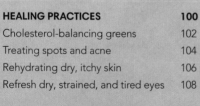
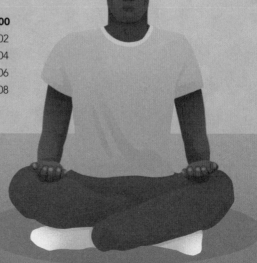

FOREWORD

Ayurveda has been flowing through my being since I was a child, and continues to help me flourish and find balance every day. Growing up in England with parents who were born and raised in India, I was fortunate enough to be exposed to much of the wisdom that many Indian people know so intimately, even before I learned to associate it with the discipline of Ayurveda.

An ancient system of healthcare that focuses on the individual rather than their symptoms, Ayurveda teaches us that in order to be completely healthy we must consider our mind, body, and spirit equally. No two people are the same, and therefore every treatment, remedy, or healing programme will be unique, and designed specifically for that person. In this way, Ayurveda makes us feel special and valued, because it "sees" us like nothing has ever seen us before.

I studied for a degree in Ayurveda more than a decade ago, and through my work as an Ayurvedic medicine practitioner, I am privileged to be able to truly "see" my clients, to help them to live well and to feel better than they ever thought they possibly could.

This little book of Ayurveda is divided into two themes. In "Wellness practices" you'll find rituals, exercises, and recipes to improve and manage your overall wellbeing; and in "Healing practices" you'll find Ayurvedic remedies and treatments that will assist you with any specific concerns you may have.

If you are completely new to Ayurveda, I hope this book will give you a taste of its potential to enhance your life, and inspire you to see that even simple changes can dramatically transform the way you feel. For those of you already familiar with Ayurvedic teachings, I hope that many of the practices you come across will demonstrate the simplicity with which Ayurveda can be joyously incorporated into your daily life.

I truly wanted this book to support you to become your own Ayurvedic practitioner, so that you may learn how to offer yourself those necessary acts of self-care that will both nurture and heal you. Take it with you wherever you go; use it as a reference point when you need it.

Enjoy exploring the life-enriching teachings of Ayurveda; my wish is that the wisdom contained within this book helps you to unlock your full potential, and to find the very best version of yourself – both now and for the rest of your life.

With love and gratitude,
Sonja Shah-Williams

INTRODUCING AYURVEDA

WHAT IS AYURVEDA?

Ayurveda is an ancient system of healthcare that focuses on treating the individual, rather than the symptoms they are suffering with. Its holistic approach means that true wellness depends on understanding each person's unique mind, body, and spiritual make-up.

Established over 5,000 years ago in India, Ayurveda offers principles and guidelines to support the mind, body, and spirit connection, as well as deep insight into the origins of the ailments we are suffering with.

PRACTICAL GUIDANCE

Ayurveda provides us with teaching tools, remedies, and rituals to manage our own health, so that we may learn to understand how foods, our lifestyle choices, the weather, the seasons, the time of day, and even our time of life affect our wellbeing.

In Ayurveda, we each have our own unique consitution type, or *prakruti*, which impacts every aspect of our lives. Living in tune with our constitution is the key to wellness and Ayurvedic practitioners can guide their clients to an even deeper understanding of their individual make-up.

CONNECTION AND BALANCE

Ayurveda is a way of thinking about the world: it is based on the beliefs that everything in the universe is connected, and that balance is the key to all that is good. Imbalance, whether in your physical body, your emotions, or your thoughts, is the cause of unhappiness and illness.

Ayurveda is also a perfect partner for modern medicine because it focuses on prevention of disease, giving each of us the know-how to take control of our own health in order to live well, for longer, and with fewer complications.

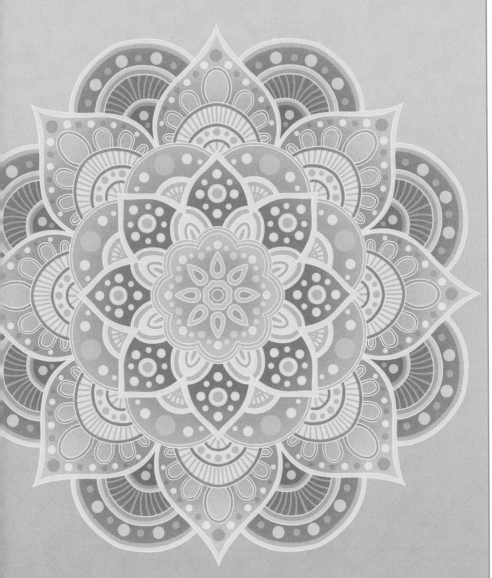

ORIGINS AND TRADITIONS

Ayurveda was born out of the wisdom of ancient Indian thinkers, and their deep desire for a better understanding of ourselves, to learn how to get the most out of our time on Earth.

WHERE IT ALL BEGAN

In the ancient Indian language of Sanskrit, *ayu* means "life" and *veda* means "knowledge": so Ayurveda is "knowledge of life". When Ayurveda originated around 5,000 years ago, it began as an oral tradition, shared by word of mouth. The knowledge is thought to have been originally acquired through deep meditation by enlightened sages (philosophers), who then passed this on to their disciples. Eventually Ayurvedic teachings were recorded in writing around 2,500 years ago, when one of the most well known Ayurvedic texts, the *Charaka Samhita*, was written. It is one of three main ancient Ayurvedic scriptures that have survived until today; along with the *Sushruta Samhita*, and *Ashtanga Hridayam*. In these texts the principles, philosophies, and practices of Ayurveda for healthy living and assessing and treating disease are recorded – these teachings remain unchanged and are those still used today.

"Ayurveda is the most sacred science of life."
(Charaka Samhita)

A SYSTEM OF HEALTHCARE

Ayurveda became recognised as a complete medicine system in India, with practitioners working as general physicians, surgeons, and specialists in specific diseases. In more recent times, Ayurveda expanded into the Western world, where it has become very popular, due in part to its focus on overall wellbeing and prevention of disease. Many complementary therapies, such as using plants to heal, and oil massage, have their roots in Ayurvedic rituals and teachings.

Though its wisdom is age-old, the principles of Ayurveda remain the same today as always, and perhaps they are even more relevant than ever in our fast-paced, modern world where the number of people afflicted by lifestyle-related problems and diseases is on the increase.

BENEFITS OF AYURVEDA

Ayurveda teaches you how to nourish your mind, body, and spirit in order to prevent the likelihood of disease, both now and into old age. By following its guidance, you not only give your body what it needs, but you can understand and manage your emotions better, which enhances your connection with yourself and others – helping you to find your place in the world. Ayurveda's guidance can be used as a reference point for everything you do, helping you to understand every aspect of your life in a deeper, more meaningful way.

STRENGTHENS THE BODY
Keeps the joints, muscles, and tissues supple, toned, and lubricated.

BOOSTS ORGAN FUNCTION
Maintains the body's organs and systems so they are able to perform key functions efficiently.

ELIMINATES TOXINS
Helps to prevent the formation and build-up in the body of ama (toxins) that can lead to disease.

**NURTURES
THE MIND**
Self-knowledge helps
you to make better
decisions, and
connect better to
yourself and others.

**AWAKENS
THE SPIRIT**
Brings a deep
understanding of
how the mind, body,
and spirit are
interconnected.

**NOURISHES
AND SUSTAINS**
Ensures the food we
eat is well digested,
for healthy tissues and
robust immunity.

AYURVEDIC BODY SYSTEMS

In Ayurveda, the body systems are described as a series of interconnecting physical and spiritual entities. Each of these must be kept in balance and good working order to achieve true holistic health.

AGNI
Our digestive fire. The quality of our digestion dictates wellness – making agni the most important aspect of Ayurvedic health.

Ojas
Biological substance in our bodies that equates to immunity. Forms when all dhatus are nourished properly.

Malas
Waste products produced by the body such as sweat, urine, and faeces.

Ama
Toxic material in the body that occurs as a result of undigested food or unprocessed emotions.

Dhatus
Our body tissues. Nourished by the foods we eat, and can be impacted by the doshas.

Prana
Our life energy, or vital life force. This energy is both physical and spiritual.

ELEMENTS AND QUALITIES
The universe is made up of five elements: ether, air, fire, water, and earth. Each element has its own characteristics, called qualities.

Srotamsi
Body channels through which life energy and substances such as blood pass.

The doshas
The three doshas are energies, each made up of a different combination of qualities, which describe its nature and role.

AYURVEDA

Pitta dosha
The dosha of transformation.

Vata dosha
The dosha of all movement.

Kapha dosha
The dosha of structure and substance.

PRAKRUTI
The unique proportion of all three doshas that makes up a person.

THE THREE DOSHAS

Each of us is made up of three doshas, or energies. When the doshas are in balance and working together, we function effectively. However, if any or all the doshas fall out of balance, disease and illness can occur.

At the heart of Ayurveda is this principle: there are five elements that make up the whole universe – ether, air, fire, water, and earth. These elements are grouped into energies, called doshas. There are three doshas – vata, pitta, and kapha – each predominantly made from a combination of two of the five elements. Their qualities are present in everything, and also in each one of us, in varying amounts. Each dosha has different properties, and the constant fluctuation of doshas' energies influences everything in the universe, including you. The balance of the doshas within you constantly changes according to a host of factors, but most people tend to have more of a certain dosha than the others. This unique constitution is known as our *prakruti*, and determines the workings of our mind, body, and spirit.

Every health problem we experience, every episode of mental or spiritual anguish, is due to an imbalance in one – or more – of the three doshas.

Getting to know the three doshas and their qualities will allow you to recognize their presence, and learn how to keep them in balance in all aspects of your life.

PITTA DOSHA
Fire and water
Pitta is the energy that governs transformation, so is responsible for functions such as digestion. Pitta has qualities that are hot, light, liquid, sharp, oily, and pungent. Its main sites within the body are the small intestine, skin, and the blood.

VATA DOSHA
Ether and air
Vata is the energy of all movement, and is responsible for functions such as breathing and circulation. Vata qualities are cold, dry, mobile, rough, subtle, light, clear, and astringent. The main sites in which it sits within the body are the colon, head, lower abdomen, and bones.

KAPHA DOSHA
Water and earth
Kapha is the energy of structure and substance and is responsible for strength in our bodies, and also our immunity. Kapha qualities are heavy, cold, slow, oily, liquid, smooth, soft, sticky, cloudy, gross, sweet, and salty. Within the body, kapha mainly sits in the lungs, stomach, sinuses, and pancreas.

THE FIRE OF AGNI

At the core of Ayurveda is agni – the body's digestive fire. Strong agni is the key to building healthy dhatus (tissues), creating immunity (ojas), and good overall health and wellbeing. When agni is weak, ama (toxins) from undigested food builds up, disrupting our bodily functions and resulting in illness.

Modern life can weaken agni: the foods we eat, being overly sedentary, and the stress we experience can all dampen our digestive fire. These principles will help you to stay mindful of your agni in daily life, keeping it strong and well-fuelled.

KEEP A ROUTINE
Eating at the same time every day means your agni knows when to expect meals, and becomes active in preparation. Agni is most active in the middle of the day, so eat your largest meal at that time.

FAST REGULARLY
Eating lightly for one day every week relieves agni and rests the digestive organs, allowing the body to rejuvenate. For more on fasting, see pages 70–71.

BE CALM
Anxiety weakens agni, so avoid eating if you are especially stressed. Eat meals mindfully, taking time and chewing food well. By giving full attention to the act of nourishment, we lend strength to agni.

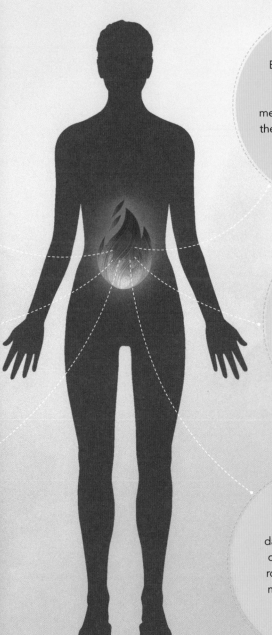

BE ACTIVE
Being too sedentary can inhibit agni. Regular exercise promotes metabolism and strengthens the entire digestive process, ensuring your food is digested fully.

EAT LIGHT
Agni can be weakened by bombarding the stomach with heavy meals and hard, cold foods. Choose light, cooked foods and stop eating before you feel too full.

AVOID THE COLD
Cold and iced drinks dampen agni, so always drink water warm or at room temperature. Too much cold or raw food can have a similar weakening effect.

THE POWER OF FOOD

In Ayurveda, food is medicine, and nutrition is at the heart of Ayurveda's philosophy. An Ayurvedic diet is full of wholesome foods that nurture our bodily functions and tissues, as well as bringing energy, joy, and clarity to our minds.

When we eat, it is the whole experience that determines how nutritious our food will be. It is crucial to understand what, why, when, where, and how to eat, so use these principles to help you:

What am I eating? Your food should be of the best quality you can afford, and in its most natural state in order to maximize the nutrients you get from it.

Where should my food come from? Food should ideally be locally and seasonally sourced, which means it will be fresher and more full of nutrients.

Which foods go together? Some food combinations produce toxins and weaken agni. Fruit, for example should be eaten on its own, as when combined with other foods the acids they create can cause indigestion. Foods with opposing qualities can also lead to imbalance.

How should my food be prepared? Too much raw food dampens the heat of our digestive fire, leading to improper digestion. Eat lightly cooked and warm foods, which are easiest for agni to handle.

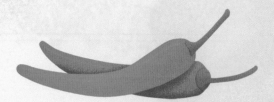

When should I eat? Aim to eat meals at roughly the same time each day, as agni's power fluctuates and different doshas dominate at different times of day.

How and where should I eat? Preparing and cooking food at home is the best way to know exactly what is in our meals. Our surroundings also profoundly effect our digestion – eating should be a pleasure, so it is important to eat at a table without distraction.

How much should I eat? Eating just the right amount means our digestion will be most effective. Overeating can cause food to remain undigested, creating ama (toxins).

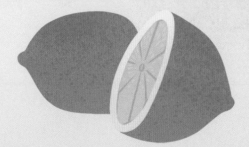

EVERYDAY PRINCIPLES

Ayurveda delivers a simple message that each of us can understand and incorporate into our daily lives – that if we follow certain daily principles, we will go a long way towards leading a holistically healthy life.

THREE MEALS
Eating three balanced and nutritious meals a day, at roughly the same time, helps agni to do its work. Fill your stomach with one third food, one third water, and leave one third empty. For ideas of what to eat and when, see pages 32–33, 46–47, and 92–93.

FIND YOUR JOY
When we take pleasure and find meaning in our lives, it benefits our mental health. For more information on how to identify and nurture those things that bring you joy, see pages 62–63.

CREATE BALANCE

"Like increases like and opposites decrease one another" refers to the qualities of the doshas, and is one of the key principles in Ayurveda that assists with diagnosis and treatment of illness. For ways to maintain balance, see pages 66–67 and 86–87.

DAILY ROUTINE

By creating a routine for yourself you work with, rather than against the doshas. Knowing when each dosha is dominant, and when agni is strongest, is key to good health. For suggestions on how to build and keep a routine, see pages 26–27.

KNOW YOURSELF

It is crucial to understand your true self so that you invite only the things and people into your life that will enhance it. Self-reflection is a powerful tool for ensuring harmony in all areas of life. For guidance on how to take time for contemplation, see pages 38–39, 42–43, and 78–79.

SLEEP WELL

If we sleep and wake according to the natural light cycles and our 24-hour body clock, we keep our bodies and minds balanced and strong. Rising early when vata is strongest, and sleeping when kapha is strongest, will ensure an energized day followed by restful sleep. For better sleep, see pages 134–135.

KEEPING
A DAILY ROUTINE

Dinacharya or "daily routine" is a guiding principle of Ayurveda as it allows you to take more ownership over your health. Each dosha's strength varies throughout the day, so to maintain balance, build your routine around the times when each dosha is strongest.

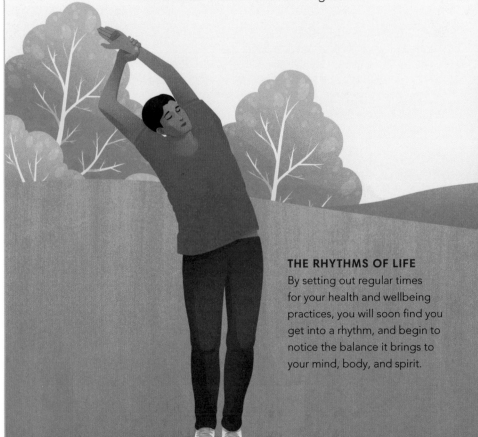

THE RHYTHMS OF LIFE
By setting out regular times for your health and wellbeing practices, you will soon find you get into a rhythm, and begin to notice the balance it brings to your mind, body, and spirit.

A GOOD LIFE

Use the following routine as a guide for how to run your day in harmony with the fluctuating power of the doshas.

01

START YOUR DAY

Early morning is when vata dosha's movement and clarity are dominant. Ideally, rise by 6am to take advantage of this time. If you are used to getting up much later, try rising half an hour earlier each day. After performing your hygiene rituals, sip warm water with a squeeze of lime to enliven your tissues. Now is also the best time for morning exercise, like yoga (see pages 34–35).

02

MID-MORNING

Kapha dosha, with its grounding earth energy, is strong now. Agni is gently awakening, so eat a breakfast that will release energy slowly, such as porridge (see pages 32–33).

03

EARLY AFTERNOON

Agni is most active at this time, fuelled by pitta dosha's heat. Aim for lunch now and make it the biggest meal of your day.

04

AFTERNOON – EARLY EVENING

Vata dosha's cold dominates once more, meaning agni is at its weakest. Keep comfortable and warm, and eat a light dinner by 7pm.

05

END YOUR DAY

Evening is kapha dosha time, when energy levels dip to prepare for sleep. Perform a calming bedtime activity, such as the massage on pages 98–99, and go to bed by 10pm. If you generally go to bed later, try retiring a few minutes earlier every night.

THE PRACTICES

WELLNESS PRACTICES

These simple self-care practices, yoga postures, rituals, routines, and recipes are designed to help you to boost your physical health, keep on top of stress and anxiety, and deepen your spiritual connection to yourself, your loved ones, and the universe.

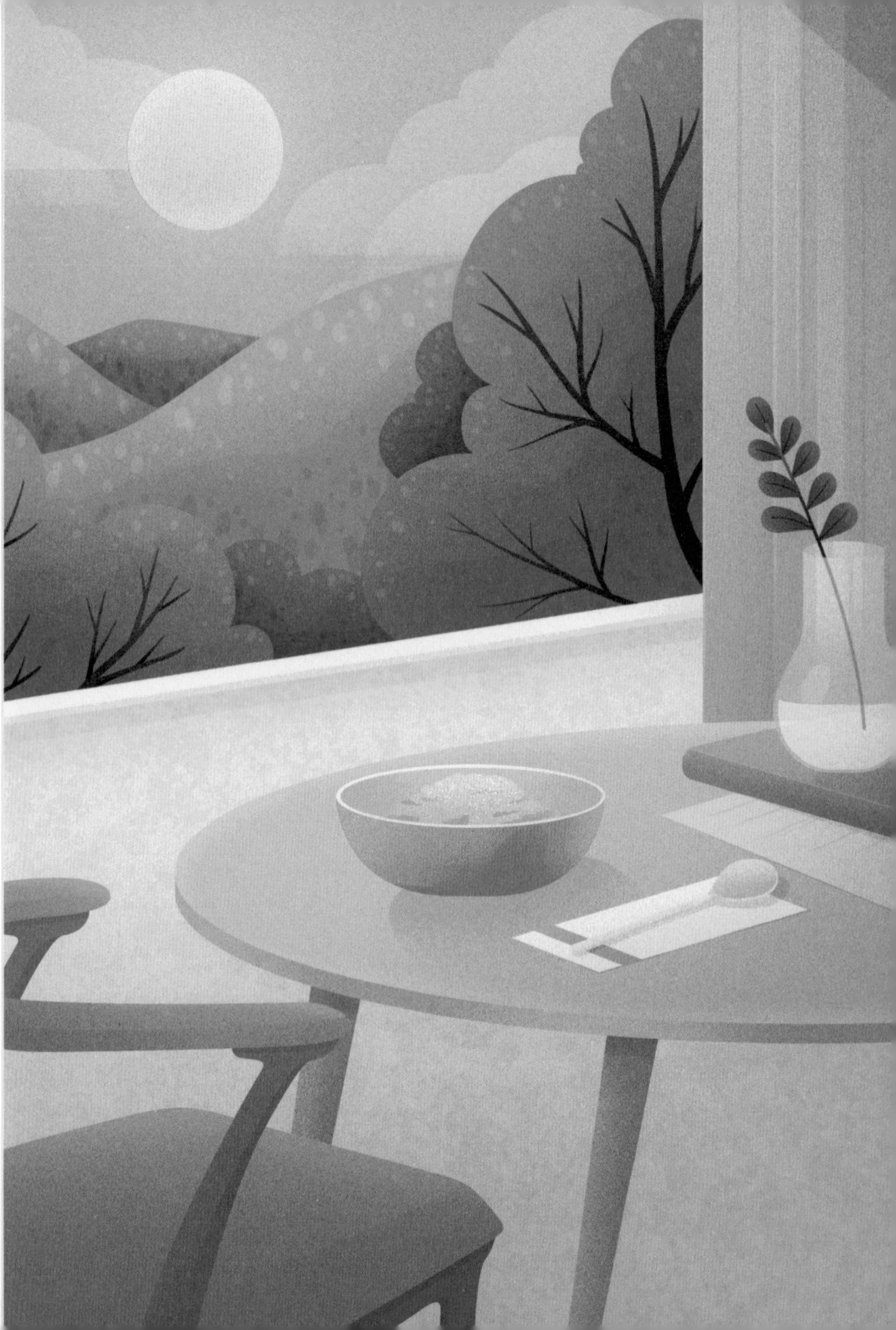

NOURISHING BREAKFAST PORRIDGE

Breakfast is important in Ayurveda because it supports the newly awakened digestive fire (agni). Porridge makes a perfect breakfast as the whole grains build strong dhatus (tissues), and release energy slowly – sustaining you until lunchtime.

NEED TO KNOW

BENEFITS Filling and well balanced – high protein and carbohydrate content; "earth" energy from oats is grounding and calming for all constitutions.

TIME 10 minutes to prepare and cook. Can be eaten every morning.

INGREDIENTS
Makes 1 serving
- 50g whole oats
- 100ml milk (or non-dairy milk)
- Large pinch each of ground cinnamon, cardamom, and nutmeg
- 1 tsp ground almonds (optional)
- Handful of raisins or chopped dried figs (optional)
- 1 tsp ghee (see pages 48–49)
- Grated jaggery (a traditional unrefined cane sugar), or raw honey (optional).

01

Put the oats and milk in a small saucepan on a low to medium heat. Add the cinnamon, cardamom, and nutmeg. Stir and cook for 5 minutes, until the oats have absorbed most of the milk and are starting to thicken.

02

Reduce the heat and add the almonds and dried fruit if using. Stir until well combined and cook for a further minute.

03

Pour into a bowl and top with the ghee, then sweeten to taste with a little grated jaggery or raw honey. Eat your porridge at a table, giving it your full attention, enjoying the warmth and nourishment it provides.

REVITALIZING MORNING YOGA

Yoga and Ayurveda are sister disciplines, often practised alongside each other for their complementary healing effects. Yoga means "union" in Sanskrit, as by moving through a range of asanas (yoga poses) you can unify your mind, body, and spirit. This short morning routine will revitalize the body and bring clarity to your mind, ready for the day ahead.

01

Table top Come to your hands and knees, legs hip-width apart, and your back flat like a table top. Hold the pose for up to a minute.

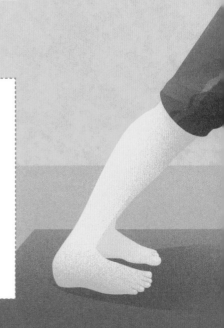

NEED TO KNOW

BENEFITS Awakens the internal organs; releases overnight stiffness and tensions; increases blood flow; balances mental and physical energy; increases mental focus; creates inner calm.

TIME Around 3–4 minutes. Ideally perform at the start of every day.

ITEMS NEEDED Yoga mat.

PREPARATION Ensure the room is warm. Wear loose, comfortable clothes.

02

Downward-facing dog From table top, tuck your toes under against the floor. Lift your knees off the ground and send your hips up and backwards to form an "A" shape with your body, keeping your arms and legs straight. Hold the pose for up to a minute.

03

Mountain From downward-facing dog, walk your hands towards your feet. Slowly uncurl to come to a standing position – back straight, arms down by your sides. Close your eyes and stay in this pose for up to a minute.

Your head hangs free in between your arms, and your gaze is towards your feet

In downward-facing dog, palms and soles of the feet are as flat against the floor as possible

TONGUE SCRAPING TO CLEAR TOXINS

Tongue scraping is an ancient Ayurvedic practice that removes toxins from the tongue, preventing illness and disease. It also enables you to enjoy your food fully throughout the day.

Most people will have some debris on the tongue in the morning, but an especially thick coating is often a sign of ama in the system. Ama is the sticky waste product of poor digestion. It builds up in the digestive tract when agni is weak, or has been overloaded by the wrong foods. If ama isn't cleared properly, it accumulates and eventually circulates around the body, finding places to settle, causing blockages in the *srotamsi* (energy channels) and unbalancing the doshas. This can lead to a condition known in Sanskrit as *Amavisha*, a chronic build up of toxins. *Amavisha* may cause a heaviness and fogginess in your mind, stiffness in your joints, and a sleepy, dull feeling after you have eaten.

AWAKENING THE TONGUE

As well as removing toxins, tongue scraping removes any lurking bacteria,

" Removing toxins from the tongue will help to prevent them re-entering the body and causing illness."

such as streptococcus, so that they do not get reintroduced into the system and cause infections. Scraping also helps to revitalize the tastebuds, by removing the coating that dulls their sensitivity.

Ideally, you should scrape your tongue every morning and evening before you brush your teeth. Use a stainless steel or copper scraper – you can buy these from any good pharmacy or health shop. Stick out your tongue and allow it to become heavy and relaxed, then scrape the surface of the tongue backwards and forwards repeatedly as you silently count to five. Rinse the scraper, then repeat. When you are finished, clean your scraper with water and allow it to dry naturally, then rinse your mouth out. Brush your teeth as normal, then drink a small glass of warm water to soothe the digestive tract.

FINDING SELF-LOVE

Ayurveda places great importance
on connecting with our true selves, and on fully learning
to love who we are. Only then will we have the capacity to
nurture ourselves well enough to achieve holistic health.

The ancient Ayurvedic message of self-love is especially relevant today when we are constantly bombarded with images and ideas of perfection, which can lead to self-criticism and low self-worth. Health problems such as anxiety and depression are often linked to these feelings, so it is crucial for our long-term wellbeing to address them. Try these simple strategies for increasing self-love:

Rise early Wisdom and inner knowledge are more readily available to us before sunrise when vata dosha's qualities of lightness, movement, and emotional sensitivity are most dominant. When we connect with these elements of vata's energy, we are able to approach ourselves with greater compassion.

Make time for yourself Taking time each day for stillness will allow you to connect to your true self more clearly. You could also try a meditation to deepen this connection (see pages 78–79).

Unplug Sensory overload can lead to excess vata dosha, which can trigger anxiety. Switch off your devices whenever possible during the day, and a few hours before bed. When you are less anxious you will be less critical and able to offer yourself more kindness.

Spend time in nature We are most healthy when we can harmonize with nature and the elements present in all three doshas. This helps to boost ojas (immunity), decreases self-criticism, and restores vital life energy (prana) – helping you discover a greater feeling of self-acceptance.

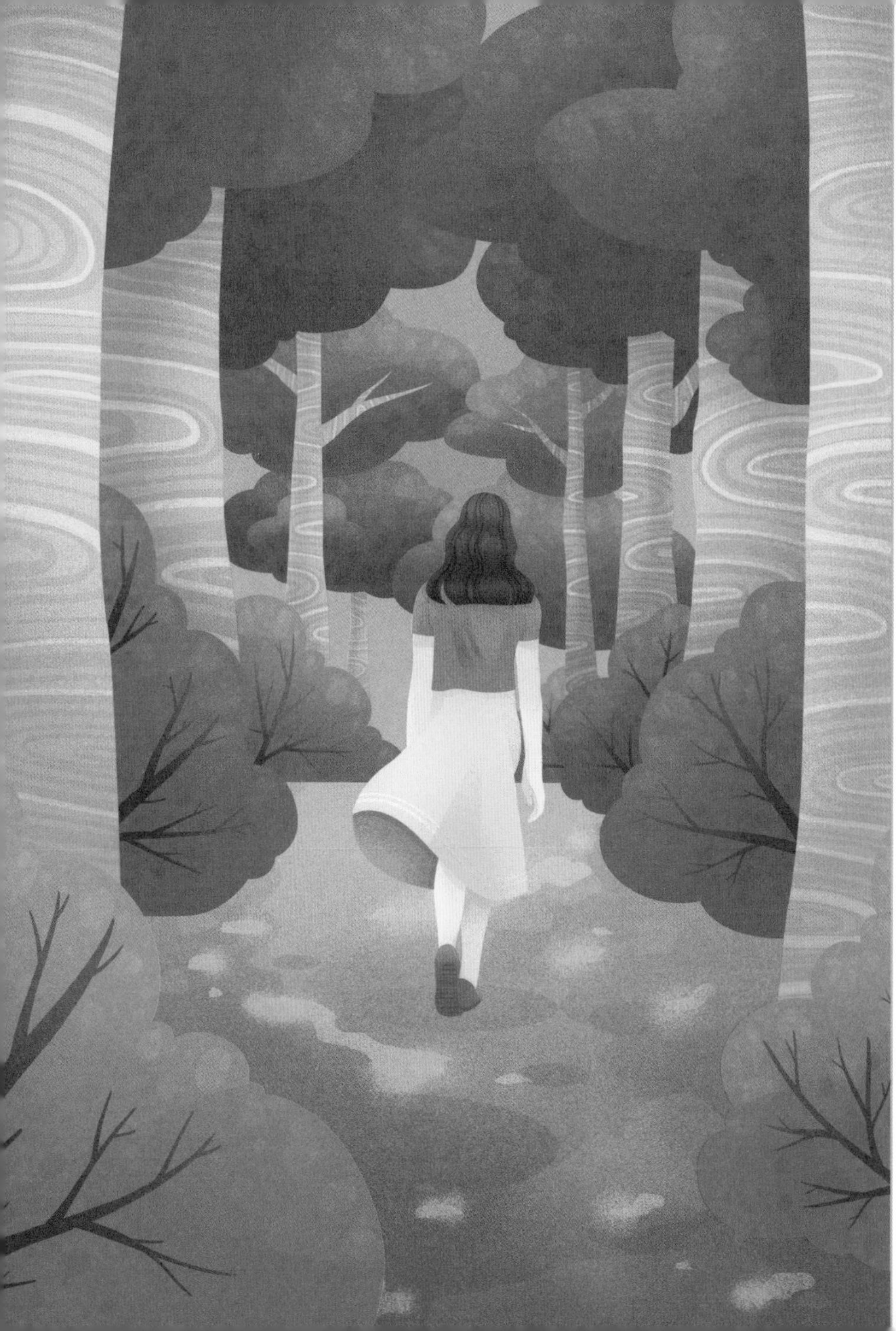

INCREASE
YOUR ENERGY

The stresses and demands of a modern, fast-paced life
mean that many of us are often left feeling fatigued and
lacking in energy. In Ayurveda, low energy is often the
result of an excess in one of the doshas.

Mental fatigue is a vata disorder, emotional fatigue is related to pitta, and physical fatigue is a kapha imbalance. If you have more of a particular dosha's qualities in your personal constitution (see pages 16–17 and 18–19), you may notice that the following typical symptoms associated with each dosha disturbance feel more pronounced.

VATA FATIGUE

Excess vata can leave you mentally drained, confused, and unable to focus.

To overcome this, eat a vata-pacifying diet that contains lots of fats and grains, as well as warm, soupy foods. Practise yoga in the evening (see pages 96–97) to calm and clear your mind; and restricting screen time will also help you stave off vata fatigue.

KAPHA FATIGUE

You will feel an overload of kapha physically – you may feel exhausted and not want to move much, and get out of breath easily when you do. To counteract

"*Balancing* whatever dosha you have an excess of with its opposing qualities will leave you revitalized."

kapha's sluggishness, aim to rise before dawn, when vata, the energy of movement, is most powerful. Cut through kapha's heaviness by eating lighter, less greasy foods such as beans, pulses, and leafy green vegetables. A morning massage with warming cedar oil (see pages 44–45 and 52–53) will also help to balance kapha's cold, dense properties.

PITTA FATIGUE

When you have too much pitta, your symptoms may express themselves in your emotions, such as finding yourself easily irritated. When you feel like this, avoid pungent and sour foods; their pitta qualities will only add to these feelings. Try journaling (see pages 66–67) to help you regulate, analyse, and manage your emotions; and massage yourself with a cooling oil (see pages 44–45 and 52–53) to cut through pitta's heat. Sip warm water infused with sweet fennel and cardamom seeds throughout the day to help temper pitta's sour qualities.

EMBRACE FORGIVENESS

The practice of forgiving yourself and others can be profoundly healing. Ayurveda teaches us that holding on to upset, or bearing grudges, can lead to a build-up of harmful ama in our bodies. This letter-writing ritual allows you the space to acknowledge, then move on from your hurt and anger – releasing any negative energy trapped in your body.

02

Use your notes to help you begin writing your letter. Try not to use negative phrases or make accusations, instead focus on describing how the situation has affected you.

01

Think about who you want to write to and why. Note down any feelings, words, or phrases that occur to you.

NEED TO KNOW

BENEFITS Lightens the burden of carrying a grudge; alleviates sadness and stress; provides a sense of relief; builds hope.

TIME Around 20 minutes, or as long as you need. Can be repeated as often as needed.

ITEMS NEEDED Paper and pen.

CAUTION You may initially feel worse as emotions are released. These feelings should pass, but if they persist, seek professional guidance and support.

PREPARATION Focus your mind by breathing slowly and deeply. Inhale through your nose for a count of 5, then exhale through your mouth for a count of 5. Repeat 3 times.

03

End your letter by offering forgiveness to the recipient. Now read your letter through, paying attention to how you feel as you do so.

04

Close the ritual by tearing up, or safely burning your letter. Visualize your negative emotions disappearing along with the words.

01

Pour a little oil into your hands and heat it by gently rubbing your palms together. Begin by massaging the oil into your neck, shoulders, and chest area in small, circular strokes using your palms and fingers.

02

Work downwards onto your arms, hands and fingers, abdomen, lower back, and buttocks. Try to keep the strokes to a smooth rhythm. If you need to, take more oil.

RESTORATIVE
SELF-MASSAGE

Abhyanga (self-massage with warm oil) is a key component of Ayurveda – nourishing the body, calming the mind, and soothing the soul. This simple massage, performed every morning before you shower, will balance your doshas and release any toxins that have accumulated overnight.

04

Sit on a towel in a chair for about 5 minutes to allow your skin to absorb the oil. Breathe deeply and slowly, inhaling through your nose and exhaling through your mouth. Shower as normal, but use only a little shower gel so as not to wash all the oil away.

03

Continue down your body, massaging the front and back of your thighs, lower legs, and the tops of your feet. Don't oil the soles of the feet, as you could slip in the shower.

NEED TO KNOW

BENEFITS Sesame oil lubricates, heals, and softens the skin and deep tissues; massage reduces tension and increases circulation; cultivates self-acceptance.

TIME 5–10 minutes, ideally every morning.

ITEMS NEEDED 3–5 tsp cured sesame oil ("curing" is a special heating process that boosts the potency of the oil); a towel.

ENJOY A
GOOD LUNCH

Make lunch your biggest, most important meal, as late morning to early afternoon is the pitta dosha time of day. Your digestion is at its strongest when pitta heat combines with the warmth of the sun to stoke the digestive fire.

Having a consistent routine for lunchtime is vital to make the most of agni when it is at its most powerful. It's not a good idea to skip lunch – if we do, we may find ourselves reaching later for sugary snacks. Their kapha properties will create heaviness and lethargy, and provide little nutrition for the dhatus (tissues).

Make ahead of time Ideally lunch should be prepared from scratch and eaten warm – cold foods are difficult to digest. You can make your meal in the morning and keep it warm in a vacuum flask until lunch time.

Boost agni Half an hour before lunch, eat a teaspoon of grated ginger mixed with a little rock salt and lime juice. Ginger digests ama, and the lime and salt kindle agni.

Don't drink too much water Drinking a lot of water can cool agni. Sip a little warm or room-temperature water with your lunch to cleanse the digestive tract and prevent ama.

Eat just enough Although lunch should be your heartiest meal of the day, it's important not to overload agni, so stop eating before you feel full.

" Grains and pulses are a great lunch option as they help to build strong tissues."

BEST FOODS FOR LUNCH

Soup A filling option, soup is easy to make and highly portable. Use a variety of vegetables and grains such as red lentils to help to build tissues. Coconut milk is rich in fats, so is good to eat when agni can digest it fully. Start with chopped vegetables and grains in a pan, and fry lightly for a few minutes. Add coconut milk, and simmer gently until the vegetables have softened and the liquid has thickened.

Chickpea curry Spices promote digestion, and fibrous chickpeas are perfect for when agni is strong. This simple curry recipe will serve one. Use oil or ghee (see pages 48–49), and fry a teaspoon of cumin seeds. Add a chopped onion, a chopped garlic clove, and 1cm of chopped, fresh ginger, and fry some more, before adding half a teaspoon each of ground turmeric, cumin, and coriander. Add 3 large chopped tomatoes and cook for 5–6 minutes before adding 250g of pre-soaked or tinned chickpeas and a good handful of fresh spinach. Add a little water and simmer for 20 minutes until the liquid has thickened.

GHEE - AN AYURVEDIC SUPERFOOD

In Ayurveda, ghee, the clarified butter of grass-fed cows, is considered medicine for both mind and body. Making your own at home is simple, and the meditative state you enter whilst preparing it is soothing for the soul.

NEED TO KNOW

BENEFITS Good for all three doshas; strengthens agni; nourishes ojas; improves joint flexibility; hydrates skin.

TIME Allow 1 hour to make. Ideally eat 3 teaspoons of ghee in a day, adding to any of your meals, for optimum health.

INGREDIENTS
Makes approx 375ml

• 500g organic, unsalted butter, cut into cubes

EQUIPMENT
Sterilized jars with screw lids, muslin cloth.

STORAGE Unopened ghee will keep for up to a year in the fridge. Once opened, keep in the fridge and use within three months.

01

Put the butter in a pan on the lowest heat setting. As the butter melts, the surface will start to bubble and foam. With a metal spoon, gently skim off this foam as it appears, but don't stir.

02

After 35–50 minutes, the milk solids will have turned brown and sunk to the bottom of the pan, leaving a clear liquid. Once the bubbles on the surface start to reduce, turn off the heat.

03

Let the ghee sit for 5 minutes before straining through a muslin cloth into a sterilized glass jar.

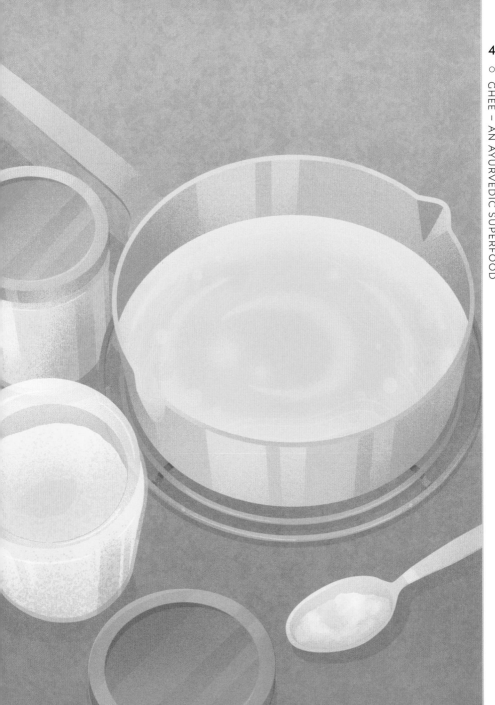

MAINTAINING A HEALTHY WEIGHT

When we feel too heavy or too light in our bodies it can be a sign that we have an excess in one of our doshas. To live our best, healthiest lives, it is important to manage our weight, and restore balance.

Excess weight is mainly caused by an imbalance of kapha dosha. Kapha and excess weight share the same qualities: heavy, slow, dense, soft, and obstructive. Being underweight may be a sign the body lacks kapha, meaning tissues are unable to develop correctly; it can also be caused by too much vata dosha, with its light, subtle properties leading to a lack of muscle mass.

Maintaining a healthy weight decreases our risk of developing certain diseases, reduces fatigue and lethargy, and boosts inner clarity and mental drive. An Ayurvedic approach isn't solely about short-term measures, but about making sustainable life choices that will have long-term benefits.

Balancing kapha dosha through your diet choices will help you maintain a healthy weight. The best foods for reducing kapha are those that are pungent, bitter, and astringent. These include chillies, leafy vegetables, and sharp green apples. Avoid meat, fast food, and processed or sugar-laden foods as these all increase kapha. If you have too little kapha, eating more dense

"Kapha dosha is associated with weight gain, so reducing it will help you maintain a healthy weight."

and nutrient-rich foods such as sweet potato, pulses, and sweet fruits, along with protein-laden light meats and fish (if you are not vegetarian) will help you to build up your tissues.

Keeping agni healthy boosts the metabolism, which helps the body to convert food into energy. A teaspoonful of grated fresh ginger before a meal will stimulate agni, helping you to avoid a build-up of ama (toxins) in the body, which can lead to weight gain. For ways to keep agni in peak condition, see pages 20–21.

An active lifestyle will also help with managing weight. Movement pacifies kapha dosha, and stimulates a sluggish metabolism. Yoga (see pages 34–35, 82–83, and 96–97) is especially good for weight management as its lightness counteracts kapha's heavy and slow qualities. Following an Ayurvedic daily routine (see pages 26–27) will also improve your metabolism and keep kapha dosha in check.

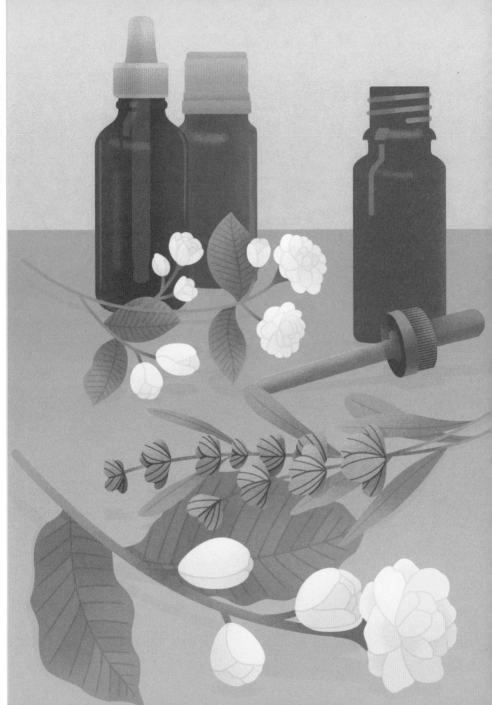

NURTURING, BALANCING OILS FOR THE SKIN

The Sanskrit word *sneha* means both "oil" and "love". When you apply oil to your body, you offer yourself love – nourishing your skin and bringing a sense of peace and contentment to your whole being.

The act of anointing the body goes back to Vedic times when plain oils and fats infused with aromatic essential oils (those naturally derived from plants and flowers) were used to to heal the body.

Essential oils have many therapeutic qualities that can bring balance to the doshas; they also penetrate deep into the dhatus (tissues), replenishing lost moisture and bringing suppleness to the skin.

Abhyanga, self-massage with oil (see pages 44–45), is a fantastic way to nurture your skin and tissues, as well as to target specific doshas. Make your own massage oils by blending essential oils with a neutral "carrier" oil, using a ratio of 1:10 in favour of the carrier, to ensure the oil is safe to apply to skin. Some essential oils are

not safe if you are pregnant, or have certain medical conditions. If in doubt, see a qualified aromatherapist.

If you feel erratic or unsettled, then you may have an excess of vata dosha. Blend cured sesame oil with grounding jasmine or lavender essential oil to soothe this instability.

If you feel quick to anger or too hot, then pitta dosha may be dominating. Blend coconut or olive oil with cooling rose or sandalwood essential oil to help temper the heat.

If you feel lethargic or stuck in a rut, it is likely you have an excess of kapha dosha. Blend mustard or flaxseed oil with warming cedar or myrrh essential oil to rejuvenate the mind and body.

COMMUNICATING
WITH OTHERS

Our emotions are our responses to particular situations or experiences. A dosha imbalance may trigger certain emotions, or may result from an emotional upset. This can impact the way we relate to, and how well we are able to communicate with others.

In Ayurveda, the more you understand yourself, the more likely you are to have balanced and fulfilling relationships. If you become familiar with the Ayurvedic qualities of your emotions, you can recognize when your communication and relationships with others may be suffering, and when you might need to take steps to correct this.

VATA IMBALANCES
If you often feel excitable or impulsive, you might have too much vata dosha.

Vata's movement may mean you find it hard to connect with those who move at a slower pace than you. **Discuss important issues** after you have eaten a meal. This will reduce the likelihood you will feel lightheaded and say something without thinking it through. **Talk about your anxieties** during the early evening when kapha's calm and grounding qualities are dominant. **Calm your restless energy** before a crucial conversation by practising alternate nostril breathing (see pages 68–69).

" *We may experience imbalance in any or all of the three doshas at some time in our relationships.* "

PITTA IMBALANCES

If you struggle with angry outbursts, this could be due to excess pitta dosha. Too much pitta can lead to perfectionism, and to being overly critical of others.

Avoid tricky discussions when drinking alcohol, or on a hot day. The added heat these bring could make you feel less tolerant of others.

Try to discuss important matters in the early evening when the temperature is usually cooler, helping to reduce the sharp tongue pitta can induce.

KAPHA IMBALANCES

If you feel insecure or hesitant to share your feelings, you could have too much kapha dosha.

Avoid discussions at bedtime which is a kapha time of day. You may fail to achieve what you set out to.

Don't make decisions after rising late – too much sleep increases kapha and this heaviness will cloud your judgement.

Try to be clear in your speech as your naturally slow pace may leave others unsure or confused about what you mean.

01

Sit on the floor or on a chair, with your back straight and hands resting on thighs. Close your eyes and take some time to observe your breath. It may be faster or more shallow than normal, which is common if you are angry or upset.

02

Now inhale smoothly through your nose – visualizing the breath flowing into your lower abdomen, mid-torso, and upper chest.

BREATHING OUT ANGER

An excess of pitta dosha can cause fiery qualities to accumulate in the mind, leading to feelings of anger. *Pranayama*, a form of breathing where you extend the breath as you inhale, then hold it before exhaling, helps to release this anger. Don't worry if you can't hold your breath for long; the more you practise, the easier it will become.

03

Continue breathing
in until you feel full of
healing, calming breath.
If you can, hold your
breath for a
count of 3.

04

Exhale gently through your
mouth, releasing the breath
gradually from your upper
chest, mid-torso, and finally
your lower abdomen.

05

Take a short pause
before repeating steps
2–4 up to 10 times, or
until you feel that your
anger has subsided.

NEED TO KNOW

BENEFITS Reduces negative emotions; regulates the
nervous system, providing a sense of calm; restores
balance to oxygen levels in the body, easing physical and
mental tension; slows a racing heart, alleviating any
associated anxiety.

TIME 5–10 minutes a day, or more as needed. Practise as
soon as you feel anger building up.

QUIETEN
YOUR EGO

The ego, or *ahamkara* in Sanskrit, is the part of our mind associated with conscious thought. We all have an ego, and like all aspects of ourselves in Ayurveda, it is important to keep it well balanced.

Our ego is responsible for our sense of self – our beliefs about our own abilities and our desires and wishes. A well-balanced and nurtured ego helps us to identify our role and importance in the world, form relationships, and create and pursue our life goals. However, if it is not kept in check, the ego can inflate, leading to vanity, stubbornness, greed, and competitiveness. An excess of pitta dosha is associated with an ego

imbalance, and can give rise to mental turmoil and agitation as the ego becomes pre-occupied with external possessions, comparisons, and self-serving behaviours. **Reducing excess pitta** from your diet can soothe any hyperactivity in the ego. Sweet, bitter, and astringent foods such as root vegetables, ginger, and beans will all pacify pitta's fiery qualities. Cooling foods are also helpful, such as whole grains, pulses, seeds, leafy greens, ghee, and

" *Reducing pitta dosha can calm the ego's negative tendencies.* "

fresh, sweet seasonal fruits. Avoid heavy meat, very spicy dishes, alcohol and tobacco as these only add to existing pitta qualities in the body.

Cultivating gratitude can help to quiet the demands of an inflated ego by focusing on what you already have, rather than the excesses the ego desires. Try writing down one thing every day that you are thankful for, no matter how big or small, to help train your ego to moderate its desires.

Small acts of kindness every day encourage you to develop compassion and empathy for others, counterbalancing the ego's tendency to selfishness. These can be practical acts, such as bringing shopping to a neighbour in need, or emotional gestures such as offering forgiveness to someone who has wronged you (see pages 42–43).

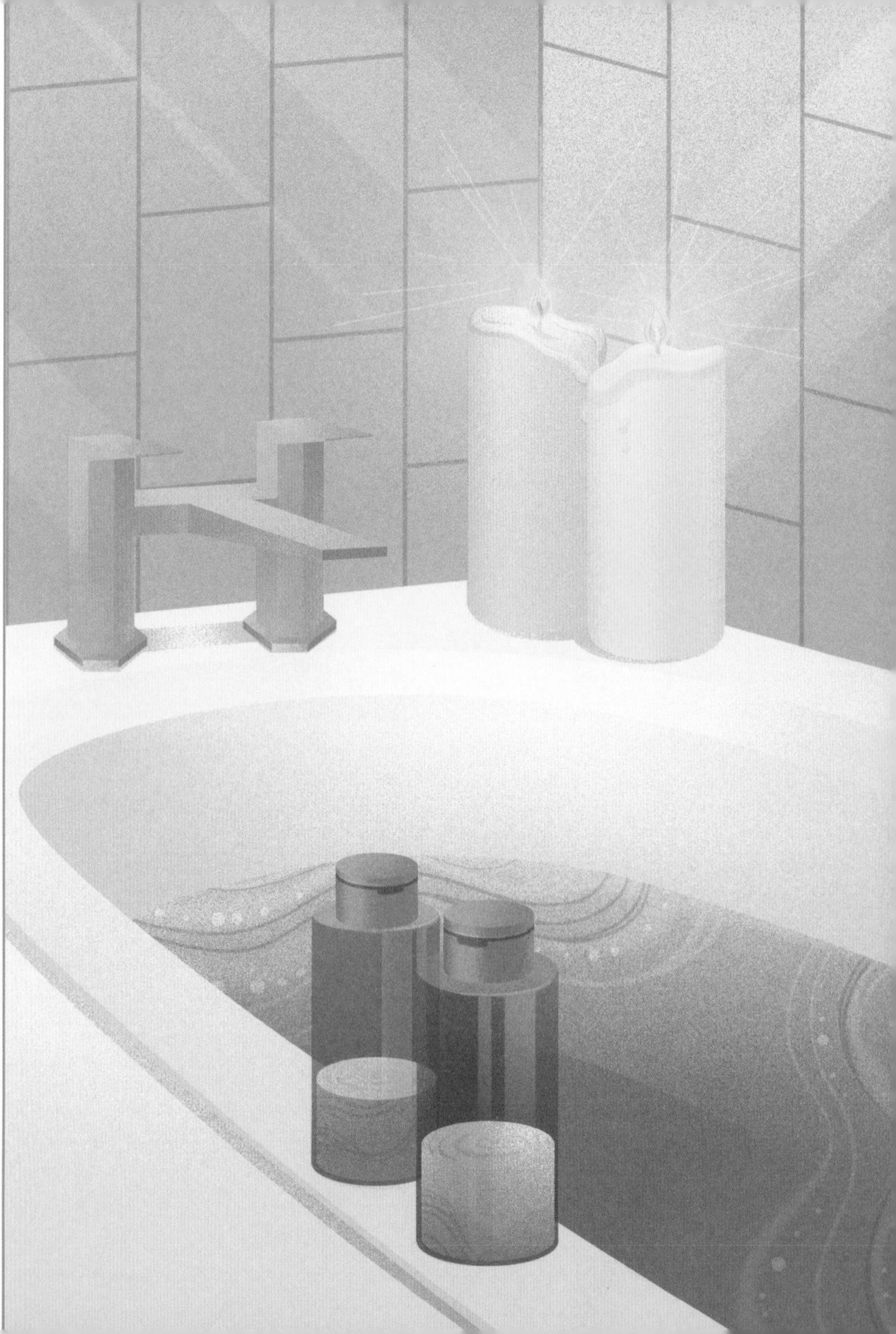

WASH AWAY YOUR STRESS

The body-heating practice of *svedana* ("to perspire" in Sanskrit) has been used by Ayurveda for centuries to treat stress. An essential-oil bath is a form of this, which can help to calm your overactive nervous system.

The body responds physically to stress, putting us on high alert. This can be a good thing, helping us to deal with emergencies, but too much for too long takes its toll, disturbing the doshas, exhausting the body and mind, and making us vulnerable to disease. We can't always avoid sources of stress, but exercises like *svedana* can reduce the symptoms when they arise.

DE-STRESSING BATH

Bathing with ginger essential oil will soothe the nervous system, improve your circulation, and flush excess stress hormones from your body as you sweat. Mix 10 drops of ginger essential oil with 2 teaspoons of jojoba oil and add to a hot bath.

To target particular emotions that may accompany stress, add the following:
If you feel anxious, you may have too much of vata's sensitivity, so add 3 drops of lavender oil.
If you feel angry, you may have too much of pitta's sharpness, so add 3 drops of rose oil.
If you feel lethargic and detached, you may have too much of kapha's heaviness, so add 3 drops of myrrh oil.

Bathe for at least 20 minutes, eyes closed, breathing slowly. Visualize the stress leaving your body through your pores. Take this type of bath twice a week, in the evenings as it promotes sleep. If you are pregnant, or have any health conditions, seek medical advice before using essential oils.

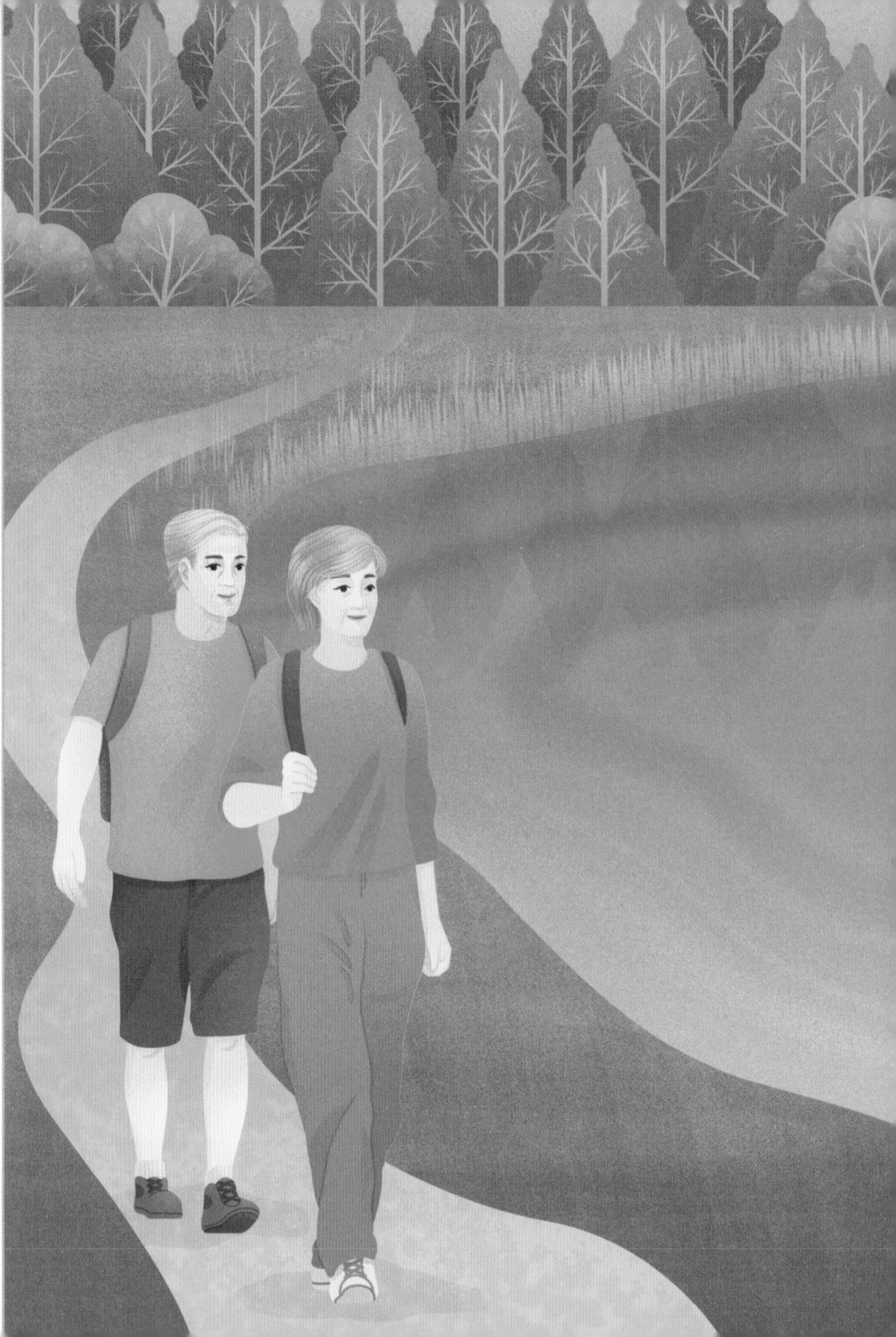

FIND YOUR JOY

In the Ayurvedic texts, holistic health is described as a state of joy that is achieved through living a fulfilled life. By identifying and doing those things that satisfy us, we can experience true health and happiness.

Joy is something every one of us can achieve. By learning to take pleasure and find meaning in every aspect of our lives, we create joy – and in turn joy creates holistic wellness. If you are struggling to identify what brings you happiness, try these techniques.

Be present Being mindful is a great way to shift your focus away from worries about the future, and to bring your awareness back to the present. Engaging fully in all you do, rather than allowing your mind to start racing ahead, will allow you to see the beauty of the task in hand. Enjoy what you feel, see, touch, smell, and hear, and truly allow yourself to find joy in even the simplest of moments.

Spend quality time with others People who have a strong, positive social network live longer and healthier lives. Socializing with friends and family increases oxytocin and dopamine, two of the body's "feel good" hormones, leaving you happy and content.

Allow for self-reflection Take time to be alone in contemplation without purpose or goals. Sit in a quiet place and simply allow yourself to observe your thoughts without making assumptions or judging them. Allowing regular time and space to explore your feelings helps to dislodge any negative emotions that may be trapped in your body. Freeing these will leave you feeling lighter and happier, helping you to achieve a true sense of joy.

BOOST YOUR IMMUNITY

In Ayurveda, ojas is the physical substance produced in our bodies that provides us with immunity and supports prana – our vital life energy. The key to building strong ojas lies in the quality of our digestion.

In Ayurvedic teachings, ojas (see pages 16–17) is crucial for us to be able to cope with the external and internal factors that can cause disease. Ojas keeps us healthy, providing us with strength, nourishment, protection, and regeneration. If digestion is weak and food is only partially processed, ama builds up, leading to unhealthy dhatus (tissues) forming. This means little ojas is produced, making the body more susceptible to illness. However, when our digestion is strong, there is no build-up of ama and our body builds healthy dhatus. This means ojas is produced, which is then circulated throughout the body, protecting our tissues, and preventing excess doshas from settling and causing disease. Healthy digestion, then, is key to the formation of strong ojas. This can be done by following the Ayurvedic principles around diet, as well as eating ojas-rich foods.

Eat cooked, organic food that's fully or mainly vegetarian to gain the nutrients you need to produce strong dhatus and

"Eating the right foods, slowly and mindfully, will lead to quality digestion and ensure ojas production."

ojas. Our body digests these foods easily, meaning ama doesn't accumulate.

Ojas-boosting foods like these easy-to-make energy balls will help to naturally boost your immunity. Soak a dried date and dried fig in a little boiled milk overnight. Remove from the milk and chop into small pieces. Heat two teaspoons of ghee in a small pan and sauté the chopped fruits for two minutes. Allow to cool, then mix in 4 teaspoons of ground almonds. Shape into three or four balls, and roll each one in roasted, desiccated coconut. Eat one or two every day.

Nourish your spirit to help you build strong ojas. Ojas forms more easily when the whole body is calm; the less stress your body is under, the less opportunity there is for toxins to build up, and for dosha imbalances to occur. Spending time with people you love, and doing activities that bring you joy, will keep your body in balance and ensure ojas forms.

JOURNALING FOR PERSPECTIVE

In Ayurveda, a balanced mind is essential to health, and it is important not to become overwhelmed by experiences and emotions. Journaling – writing, observing, and processing your thoughts – will help you maintain a sense of perspective.

NEED TO KNOW:

BENEFITS Creates space for calm, objective reflection; increases self-awareness.

TIME 10–15 minutes. Ideally practise once a day, but more if you wish.

ITEMS NEEDED Journal or notebook; pen.

PREPARATION Find a quiet space to sit comfortably. Focus your mind by breathing slowly and deeply. Inhale through your nose for a count of 5, then exhale through your mouth for a count of 5. Repeat 3 times.

01

Begin with gratitude: write down all the things you are thankful for today. Don't think too much about what to write, just note your thoughts as they occur to you.

02

Now write down anything else that has affected you since you last wrote. What have you achieved? What would you like to achieve tomorrow? Try to use positive words and phrases if you can.

03

When you are ready to finish, take a moment to read over and reflect on what you have written. Give thanks for this opportunity to explore your feelings, before closing your journal.

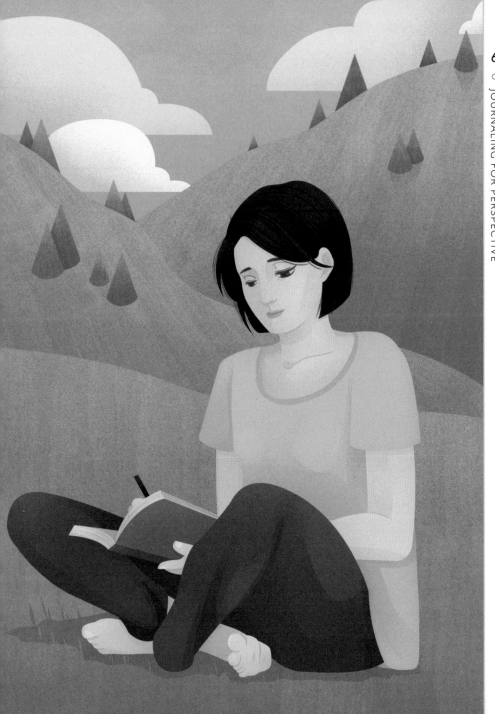

BREATHING FOR FOCUS

Alternate nostril breathing (*anuloma viloma*) is an ancient technique used in Ayurveda to help awaken prana – our vital life force. Perform this simple exercise at the start of your day to bring nourishing oxygen into your body, clear your energy channels (*srotamsi*), and revitalize the mind to begin your day with focus.

02

Slowly exhale all the air in your lungs through your left nostril. Now inhale slowly, until the lungs feel full again.

01

Use the thumb of your right hand to press against and close your right nostril.

NEED TO KNOW

BENEFITS Calms the nervous system; improves lung capacity; improves concentration; creates a feeling of positivity and harmony; allows energy to flow freely.

TIME Around 5 minutes, ideally every morning.

ITEMS NEEDED Yoga mat, or straight-backed chair.

PREPARATION Sit on your mat cross-legged, or in a chair with your back straight.

CAUTION If you experience chest pain, dizziness, or discomfort, stop immediately and return to normal breathing. Don't attempt this exercise if you have recently undergone surgery.

03

Simultaneously release your thumb from your right nostril and close your left nostril with your right ring finger. Slowly exhale all of the air in your lungs through your right nostril.

04

Slowly inhale, then release your ring finger from your left nostril and close your right nostril with your thumb. Exhale slowly through your left nostril. This completes one round.

05

Repeat for up to 10 rounds. To finish, remove your finger and thumb from your nose and allow your breathing to return gradually to normal.

Left nostril is covered with right ring finger as you exhale through right nostril

Rest your left hand palm-up on your left knee

FASTING TO CLEANSE AND CLARIFY

In Ayurveda, fasting helps to remove ama from the body by providing agni with the opportunity to rest and recharge. By reducing heavy foods from your diet, you can cleanse your system, as well as improve your ability to concentrate and experience clarity.

In a world where we are constantly on the go, many of us have become accustomed to eating as and when we want, rather than when we are truly hungry. This can lead to agni becoming overloaded, an accumulation of food in the digestive tract, and ama forming. Fasting has been part of Ayurvedic teachings, as well as in wider Indian culture, for millennia. According to the ancient Hindu texts, fasting is also undertaken in order to focus on spiritual reflection, as when

we restrict what we eat, we leave space for clear thinking. Talk to your doctor before fasting, especially if you have specific health issues. Don't fast if you are pregnant, breastfeeding, or underweight.

HOW TO FAST
Start slowly It is a good idea to introduce fasting gradually – start by replacing all your meals one day a week with, for example, a small bowl of khichdi (see pages 92–93) three times a day. Leave

"Fasting gives your body and mind the opportunity to restore and replenish."

3–4 hours between each meal, and don't eat after 7pm, when agni is at its weakest. Try to pick the same day each week for your fast; this way your digestive system knows when to expect a break.

Replace one meal Once you have become accustomed to your weekly cleanse, try replacing your breakfast khichdi with a small bowl of chopped, ripe, sweet fruits such as red apples, black grapes or nectarines. Fruits are light and will further allow your digestive fire to recuperate. Try not to see fasting as denying yourself food, but rather as a way of providing your body with the time it needs for healing. Break your fast gently by adding some cumin seeds fried in a little oil and a portion of leafy greens to your evening khichdi.

Drink plenty of hot water Drinking hot water while cleansing will help to clear undigested food from the gut. If fasting leaves you feeling nauseous, add a little lemon juice – it will soothe your stomach.

02

Close your eyes and relax your facial muscles. Take a minute or so to become aware of how you feel right now, in your mind and body.

01

Lie or sit on a yoga mat, or sit in a chair. If lying down, place your palms flat against your abdomen, index fingers and thumbs touching. If sitting, rest your hands, palms up, in your lap.

MANTRA TO NURTURE SELF-ESTEEM

Mantras are repeated phrases that re-energize the mind and replace negative thoughts with positive ones. In this simple ritual, you can grow your self-confidence using the Sanskrit mantra *So Hum* which means "I am that" – affirming that you are one with the universe, protected by its unconditional support.

04

Now exhale slowly through your mouth for a count of 3 while silently saying "*Hum*". Repeat the mantra for up to 10 minutes, breathing in on "*So*", and out on "*Hum*".

03

Take a slow, deep breath in through your nose for a count of 3 while silently saying "*So*". Focus only on the word of the mantra.

05

Finish by bringing your awareness to how you now feel; you may notice any negative thoughts have dissipated, and that you feel more positive and confident.

NEED TO KNOW

BENEFITS Reduces vata dosha, calming overstimulation in the mind; promotes self-love and self-acceptance; separates the true self from negative thoughts.

TIME 5–10 minutes, or more if needed. Ideally practise every day to strengthen and cultivate self-confidence.

ITEMS NEEDED Yoga mat, or chair with supportive back.

PREPARATION Wear loose, comfortable clothing and perform on an empty stomach.

BE FULLY PRESENT
IN YOUR LIFE

At times we are all distracted, whether by external sources like TV, or our own minds that stop us from being fully present. By bringing in the stabilizing qualities of kapha dosha, we can slow our thoughts and focus deeply, bringing balance to our internal world, and allowing us to connect better to the outer world.

NEED TO KNOW

BENEFITS Creates stillness and reconnects you to the present; prevents distraction from unhelpful thoughts; increases concentration and self-awareness; calms the nervous system.

TIME Around 10 minutes or more if needed. Try to practise this visualization every day.

PREPARATION Sit comfortably in a chair with your back straight and your shoulders relaxed. Place your hands in your lap, close your eyes, and take a moment to allow your breathing to slow.

01

Picture a perfect sunny day. You are looking out over a stretch of gently bobbing water, surrounded by beautiful, thriving trees and flowers.

02

Now visualize yourself sitting in a wooden boat on the water. Enjoy this idyllic place, silent apart from the birds above you, and the water softly lapping at your boat.

03

Smell the clean, fresh air, feel the sun on your face, and the gentle breeze on your skin. Keep this scene in your mind, noticing all the sights, smells, and sounds, for around 10 minutes before gently bringing yourself back to the present.

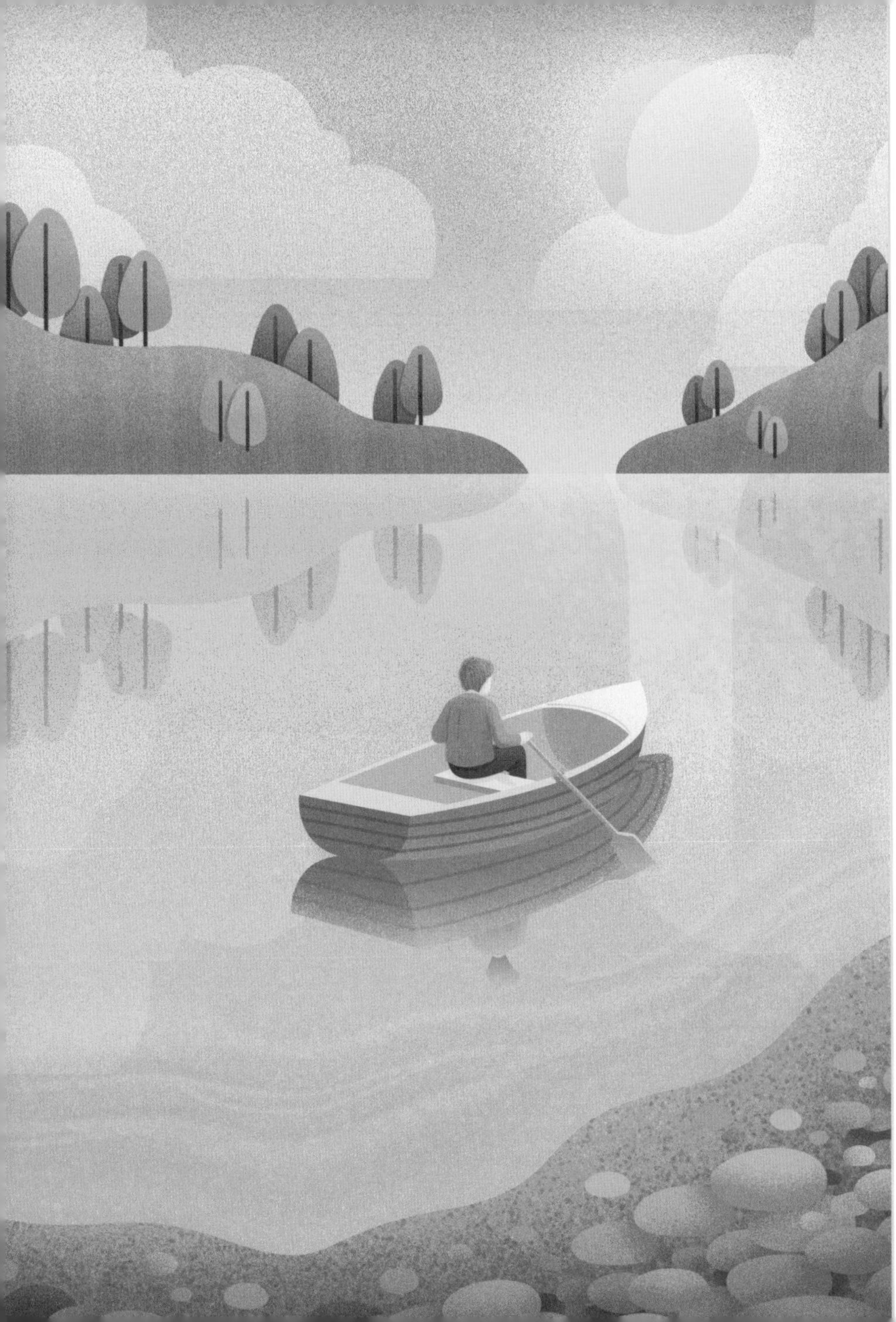

PREPARING FOR CONCEPTION

Bringing a baby into the world is a joyful and important decision for many of us. Ensuring holistic wellness and balance in all areas of your life is the key to conceiving successfully.

In Ayurveda, the preparation period, around six months before you become pregnant, is just as vital as the pregnancy stage itself. By following these principles, both men and women can ensure their mind, body, and spirit are in peak condition for making a baby.

Improve your reproductive tissue (*shukra dhatu*) quality with the right nutrition. A ripe banana with ghee has kapha properties, building sturdy tissues in both men and women. Heat a teaspoon of ghee in a small pan, add a sliced, ripe banana, and stir to coat with the ghee. Cinnamon is also good for removing toxins, so add a pinch of ground cinnamon before serving. Eat as a mid-morning snack an hour after breakfast, and two hours before lunch.

Take a bath in ashoka, a powerful Ayurvedic remedy made from the bark of an Indian tree. Known as the "remover of sorrow", it is particularly linked to female health, reducing physical pain in

"*Harmony in all elements of the mind, body, and spirit is essential for conception.*"

the reproductive organs. If you are trying to conceive, boil three tablespoons of ashoka powder in two cups of water until the amount has reduced by half. Add this to your bath every night. You can buy ashoka from health food shops.

Take rejuvenating chyawanprash, an Ayurvedic jam-like remedy that contains Indian gooseberry, which is rich in vitamin C, helping to nourish reproductive tissues and build ojas. Boil a glass of milk and stir in a teaspoon of jam. Allow to cool a little before drinking. Drink each night whilst trying to conceive. You can buy chyawanprash from Indian food shops.

Ensure you get enough quality sleep to keep your body systems functioning properly – this is especially helpful for ensuring predictable monthly menstrual cycles. Follow your natural circadian rhythm (24 hour sleep/wake cycle) by going to bed no later than 10pm, and avoid anything stimulating, such as digital devices, two hours before bed.

MEDITATION FOR MINDFULNESS

Meditation teaches us how to create silence within, freeing us from any unhelpful thoughts. This mindful practice anchors you to the present by focusing your attention on your breathing – helping you to resist distractions. Use it to bring a sense of calm and clarity to your entire being.

02

Take a slow, deep breath in through your nose for a count of 3. Notice the rise of your chest, as the breath fills the spaces in your body.

01

Close your eyes and start to notice any thoughts you have. Allow them to pass through your mind without judging or analysing them.

NEED TO KNOW

BENEFITS Promotes compassion, tolerance and understanding; helps to overcome mental resistance and agitation; enhances the mind, body, and spirit connection; calms the nervous system.

TIME At least 5 minutes. Ideally perform every morning or evening, on an empty stomach.

ITEMS NEEDED Firm cushion or straight-backed chair.

PREPARATION In a quiet space, sit in a chair or cross-legged on a cushion on the floor, hands resting on your legs, with palms up.

03

Exhale through your mouth for a count of 3, focusing only on the fall of your chest as your breath leaves the body. Continue breathing and observing in this way for at least 5 minutes.

04

Finish by bringing your awareness back to the present. Take a moment to give thanks for the opportunity to connect with your true self, before opening your eyes.

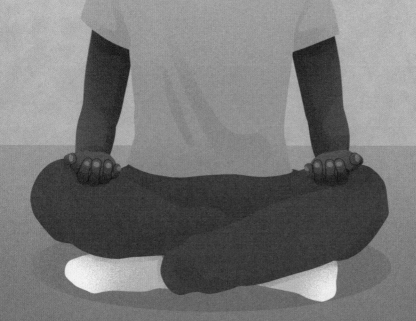

Shoulders are relaxed

Neck and spine are aligned

SPEAK YOUR TRUTH

It is important for our mind, body, and spiritual health to connect fully to our true selves. The chakras (Sanskrit for "wheels"), and the throat chakra especially, play a key part in helping you to communicate your truth.

The ancient Hindu concept of the chakras states that there are seven locations in the body through which prana (energy) flows. Each chakra has a colour that it responds to, which can bring healing properties to this location. When our chakras are fully open and in alignment, we feel holistically well and connect strongly with our true selves.

Vishuddhi, the throat chakra, is the fifth chakra, responsible for our communication, creativity, and self-expression. The colour blue is associated with *vishuddhi,* as it is believed to represent truth and wisdom.

UNBLOCK *VISHUDDHI*
If you are suffering with anxiety and low self-esteem, constantly on the edge of voicing your feelings, but fearful of being judged, then *vishuddhi* may be blocked. You may have a stiff neck, sore throat, or struggle to clear your throat. In order to speak your truth you need to unblock the throat chakra, so energy can flow freely.
Throat massage Lubricating the tissues with oil will reduce tension in the muscles, clearing any blockages. It is also a way to offer love and compassion to your voice,

_"Unblocking the throat chakra
will help to rid you of fears about
speaking your truth."_

helping you to express yourself more clearly. Coat both hands with a little cured sesame oil and use finger pads and palms to massage your throat with smooth, alternate, upward strokes from collarbone to chin.

Truth affirmation _Sat Nam_ is a powerful Sanskrit affirmation that means "truth is my identity". By focusing on these words you help your entire being to absorb this positive message, the energy of which will unblock _vishuddhi_. Stand in front of a mirror, close your eyes, and imagine your reflection is surrounded by healing blue light. Slowly say _Sat_ (to rhyme with "but"). Visualize the word moving from your navel to your heart, and then into your throat. Now say _Nam_ (to rhyme with "palm"). Again, follow the word from your navel to your heart, and into your throat. Repeat the phrase for five minutes, before slowly opening your eyes and smiling at your reflection.

ENERGIZING AFTERNOON YOGA STRETCH

Mid-afternoon is often when we feel stiff from sitting at our desks, or low in energy after lunch. This simple routine is ideal for a work break, and will boost your energy naturally by increasing blood flow to vital organs and tissues.

NEED TO KNOW:

BENEFITS Aids digestion; stretches the spine, hips, and limbs; improves oxygen supply to the brain, re-energizing the mind.

TIME Around 5 minutes. Every afternoon, at least half an hour after eating.

01

Standing back bend Stand with feet together, palms against your lower back, and elbows bent. Gaze up and lean back. Hold for 15 seconds, gently breathing through your nose, then return to your starting position and relax. Repeat 3 times.

02

Left side stretch With feet together, reach your arms up and grab your left wrist with your right hand. Pull on your wrist as you lean to the right and push your hips to the left. Hold for 15 seconds then return to centre. Repeat 3 times.

03

Right side stretch Repeat step 2 on your right side, holding your right wrist with your left hand, leaning left and pushing your hips right. Hold for 15 seconds. Repeat 3 times.

In left side stretch, grip the left wrist with your right hand, and lean to your right

Keep feet together and legs strong as you send hips to the left

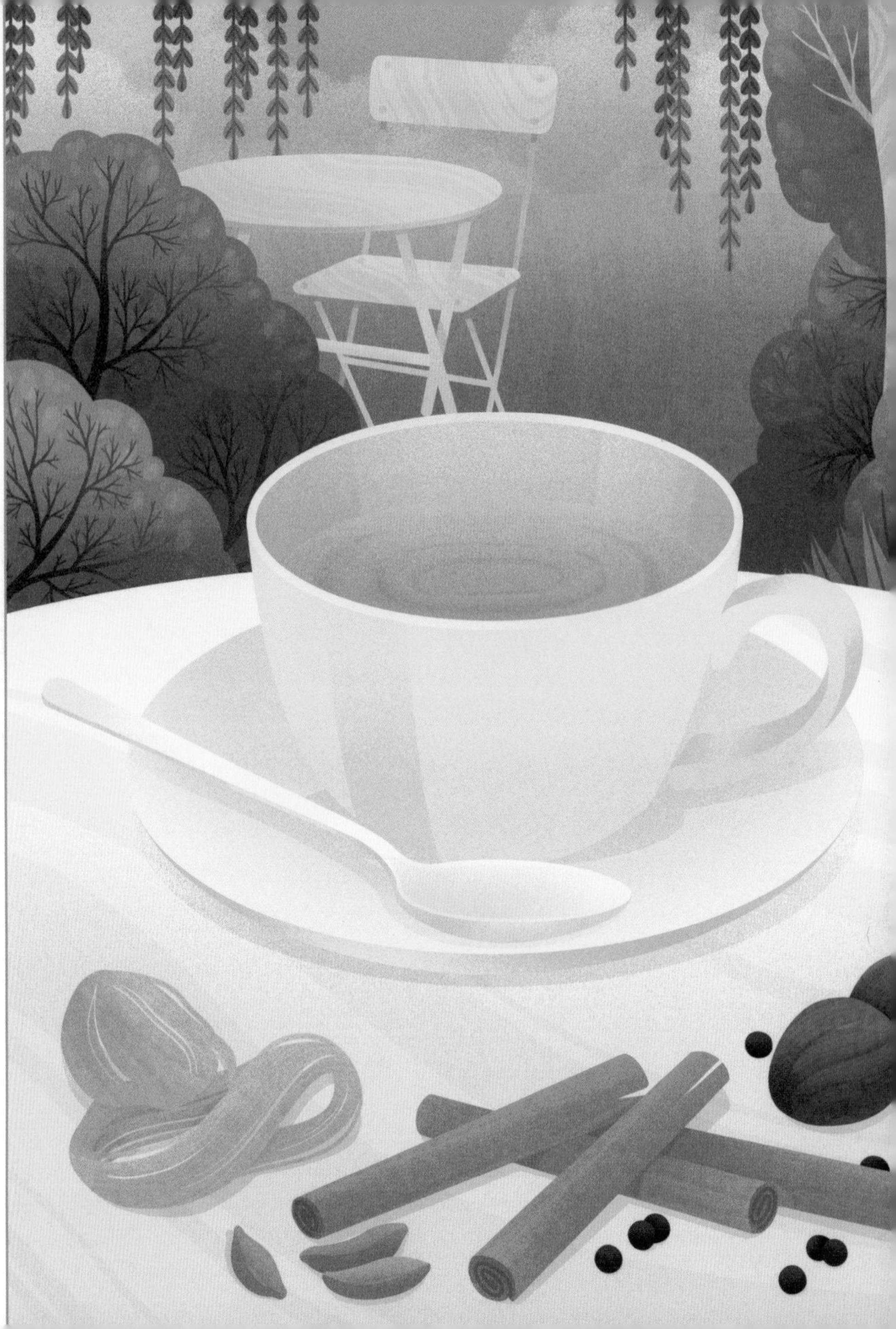

REVIVING MASALA CHAI

Chai is the Indian word for tea and masala chai is a traditional tea made with spices, water, and milk. A popular drink in every Indian household, it boosts agni, increases energy, and enhances the body's immunity.

NEED TO KNOW

BENEFITS Clears ama (toxins); balancing for all three doshas.

TIME Spice blend: about 25 minutes; chai: about 5 minutes.

INGREDIENTS

Spice blend makes approx 50 teaspoons; chai serves 2

- Masala spice blend: 12g green cardamoms; 12g cloves; ½ a nutmeg, grated; 25g cinnamon sticks; 50g dried ginger, cut small; 6 black peppercorns; 1 mace flower
- 225ml cold water
- 1 tsp loose black tea leaves
- 70ml milk (or non-dairy milk)
- Jaggery/brown sugar to taste

EQUIPMENT Spice or coffee grinder, or pestle and mortar

STORAGE Masala spice blend can be stored in an airtight jar in a cool, dry place, for up to 6 months.

01

To make the masala blend, roast the spices in a pan over a medium heat for 10–15 minutes, stirring constantly. Allow to cool, grind to a fine powder (in batches if necessary) and sieve to remove any larger bits that remain.

02

Put the water in a saucepan on a medium heat and add ⅓ teaspoon of masala blend. When it boils, add the tea leaves, stir well, and reduce the heat to a simmer for a minute.

03

Add the milk and simmer for another minute before turning off the heat. Strain the tea into a pot to serve, and sweeten with jaggery or sugar if you wish.

NURTURING WISDOM

In Ayurveda, good health is achieved through balancing our mind, body, and spirit. If you find yourself constantly unwell or out of sorts, this could be your body's way of telling you that the balance has tipped somehow, and that you need to exercise wisdom to restore this.

Prajnaparadha is a Sanskrit term meaning "an assault against wisdom". It refers to when we know we are doing something that may be bad for us, but we do it anyway. For example, we may understand that certain foods make us feel unwell, but we still eat them. Similarly, we know that emotions such as hate, greed, anger, jealousy, and envy can drain our mental reserves, but at times they still consume us.

Ayurveda teaches us that we were all endowed with reason and have the potential to engage in a higher level of thinking that goes beyond the instant gratification of our earthly desires.

When we exercise this reason, and nurture our wisdom, we bring balance to our mind, body, and spirit. This helps us to achieve a more significant sense of peace and contentment, and to experience better all-round health.

"Seeking the very best version of yourself through selflessness can bring balance to your whole being."

ACTS OF KINDNESS

If we are able to live with an awareness of *prajnaparadha*, we can move beyond any limiting behaviours and find balance. One way to do this is to undertake acts of kindness that are totally selfless, with no expectation of anything in return. Even if you can only find time once a week, you will feel the benefit in your life. You could volunteer for a charity you feel an affinity with, or simply help a neighbour who may need some practical or emotional support. Make sure you fully engage in the act of kindness as you do it. Make an effort to get to know and understand your neighbour as a person, or to learn about the work the charity you are supporting undertakes. This will make it more rewarding for you as well as fostering compassion and understanding of others, both of which nurture wisdom.

FACIAL MASSAGE ROUTINE

Massaging your face with oil keeps skin supple and stimulates energy centres on the face called *marma* points. This allows free flow of energy through the body's *srotamsi*, or channels.

NEED TO KNOW

BENEFITS Relieves stress; clears toxins; improves the look and elasticity of facial skin and muscles.

TIME About a minute for each step. Ideally, perform every evening before bed on cleansed skin.

ITEMS NEEDED Teaspoon of sesame oil.

PREPARATION Sit comfortably in a warm place, such as your bedroom.

Arrows indicate the direction of strokes

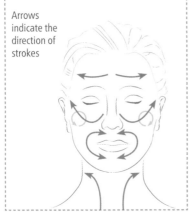

01

Pour oil into your hands and rub together to warm the oil. Place your fingers at the centre of your forehead and stroke outwards, one hand after the other.

02

Still alternating hands, stroke from the sides of the nose, over the cheeks to each temple. Press gently on the temples for a few seconds. Then make circular movements over your cheeks.

03

Place two fingers horizontally under your nose, then trace them around your mouth to meet at the chin, and back to the starting point.

04

Finally, use your palms to make upward strokes on your neck, alternating your left and right hands.

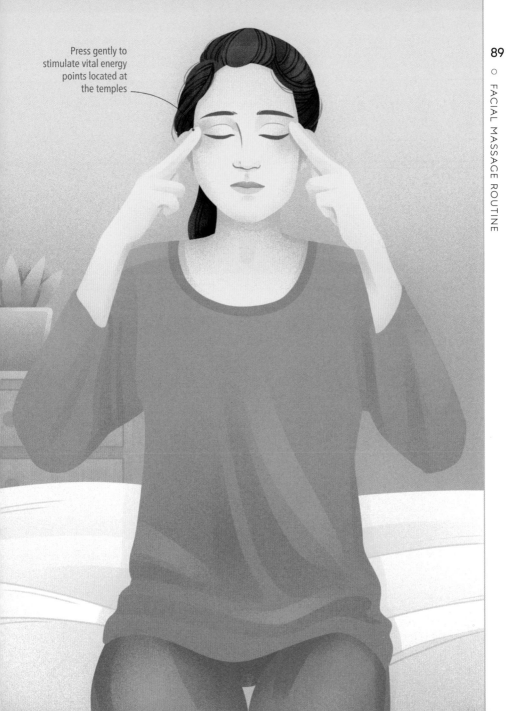

Press gently to stimulate vital energy points located at the temples

KEEP JOINTS SUPPLE

In Ayurveda, joint pain arises from an excess of vata dosha and its cold, dry, and brittle qualities. Without enough lubrication, joints rub together as they move. Reducing excess vata willl relieve the pain and inflammation this causes.

Joint pain is something we all experience at some time or another. Our joints are subject to natural wear and tear as we age, as well as being affected by stresses and strains brought on by exercise or injury. When you experience pain and inflammation in your joints, it is likely you have been aggravating vata dosha. This can be from eating too many cold, dry foods that are difficult to digest; or from over-exercising, overworking, or feeling stressed, all of which can increase vata.

Decreasing vata Stick to a daily routine (see pages 26–27) – vata craves routine in order to keep its flighty and erratic qualities in check. Intense exercise produces excess vata, which will further stress your joints. Opt instead for brisk walks, light yoga, or swimming. Keep your stress levels down (see pages 60–61), and eat foods that are unctuous (rich in good fats) to lubricate the joints, and warm and lightly spiced to temper vata. Drink hot water with a pinch each of cinnamon, turmeric and ginger powders, as these spices all reduce vata.

"*Eating a diet rich in fatty acids counteracts the dry qualities of vata that cause joint pain.*"

Reducing inflammation Essential fatty acids such as omega 3 and omega 6 help to regulate the body's immune response, so can reduce inflammation, and also keep joints supple by oiling them. If you eat fish, be sure to include mackerel, sardines, trout, or salmon, in at least three meals a week. Plant-based foods high in omega 3 and 6 include legumes, pulses, grains, nuts, seeds, cereals, leafy greens, and soya products. Eggs and ghee are also great sources of essential fatty acids.

Mustard oil massage Massaging painful joints with warm oil will relieve inflammation by nourishing the joints and tissues, stimulating movement, and increasing blood flow. Mustard oil, which you can buy in health food shops, is especially heating, so will counteract the coldness of vata. Every day after bathing, while your skin is still warm and slightly damp, gently massage 1 teaspoon of mustard oil into affected joints.

BALANCING EVENING MEAL

According to Ayurveda, our evening meal should be the smallest and lightest of the day. This is because agni is least active at this time, and would struggle to break down heavier foods. Khichdi, a traditional Indian dish of mung beans and basmati rice, is both easy to digest and balancing for all doshas.

NEED TO KNOW:

BENEFITS Good source of protein and rich in multi-nutrients; quick and easy to digest; detoxifies the intestines and liver.

TIME 15 minutes for preparation and cooking. Ideally, eat at least 3 hours before you go to bed.

INGREDIENTS
Makes 1 serving

- 45g basmati rice
- 25g mung beans
- 140ml of cold water
- Large pinch of turmeric
- Pinch of salt
- 2 tsp ghee (see pages 48–49)

VARIATION If you like strong flavours, fry a teaspoon of cumin seeds, a few slices of garlic, and 4–5 curry leaves in the ghee. Add to cooked khichdi and mix well.

01

Place the rice and mung beans in a sieve or strainer and rinse thoroughly under warm, running water. Put the rice and beans in a saucepan and top with the cold water.

02

Add the turmeric and salt, and stir well. Bring the pan to boil, then reduce the heat and simmer gently. Put a lid on the pan, leaving a gap for steam to escape.

03

After 10 minutes, the water should have evaporated. If not, cook for a further 2 minutes. Once ready, spoon the khichdi into a bowl, top with the ghee, and serve immediately.

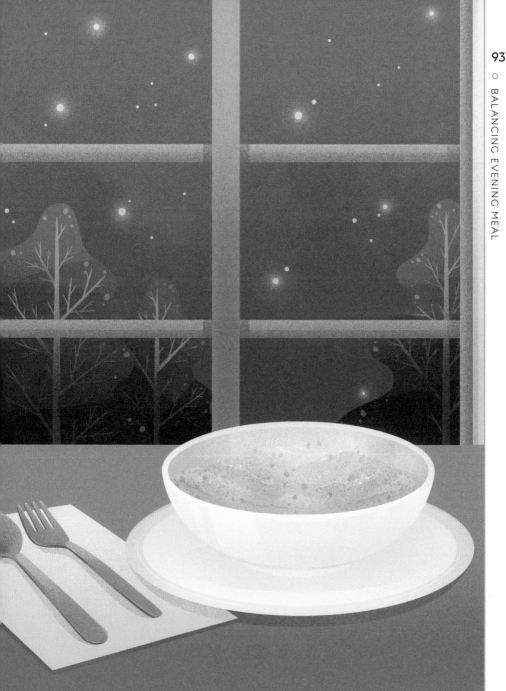

LIVE WELL,
AGE WELL

By following simple Ayurvedic principles and making the
best lifestyle choices, we can meet the challenges of
adapting to the different phases of life and enjoy the
best of health as we grow older.

Ayurveda categorizes the stages of our
lives according to the three doshas: childhood
represents kapha and a period of slow, stable
growth; adulthood embodies the warm,
quick, and transformative properties of pitta;
and old age represents the lightness, dryness,
and wisdom of vata.

By preparing for increased vata, we can
reduce our likelihood of developing age-
related ailments and ensure our later years
are as joyful as possible – a time where we
can truly relish the additional insight and
clarity that comes with enhanced vata.

AYURVEDIC AGEING

A balanced diet Stick to the Ayurvedic
principles of nutrition (see pages 22–23) to
avoid overburdening your digestive system,
which can lead to premature ageing. As you
get older, you need to ensure you drink
more water each day to counteract vata's
dryness and keep your tissues strong.

Daily routine Known as *dinacharya* (see
pages 26–27), this is one of the key
principles of Ayurveda. The repetitive
nature of these rituals also helps to keep
your brain active and strengthen memory.

"An Ayurvedic lifestyle ensures the process of growing older is as comfortable and enjoyable as possible."

Sleep well If you go to bed and rise in line with your natural bodily rhythms (the 24 hour sleep/wake cycle) you will sleep better. Good quality sleep is especially important as you get older, because poor sleep can cause a stress response in your organs, impairing their functioning, leading to illness and premature ageing. Make sure you go to bed at the same time each night, and try some of the techniques on pages 134–135 beforehand to ensure you get a sound night's sleep.

Apply warm oils *Abyhanga*, self-massage with warm oil (see pages 44–45), will counteract vata's dry properties, and keep your skin and deeper tissues nourished. This can be especially helpful for those living with conditions such as Parkinson's and Alzheimer's disease, as massage reduces the production of stress hormones, and increases blood circulation to the brain, slowing the deterioration of brain cells. See pages 98–99 for a detoxifying scalp massage ritual you can try before bedtime.

YOGA FOR SOUND SLEEP

By the end of the day, our minds and bodies are often overloaded and overstimulated. Yoga is an effective way to wind down, and certain asanas are especially useful for promoting sleep. These simple poses will help to quiet your mind and release tension from your body, ready for a good night's rest.

01

Legs up the wall On a yoga mat or towel, lie on your back near a wall, arms by your sides. Place your legs up the wall to form an "L" shape with your body. Hold for up to 2 minutes.

NEED TO KNOW

BENEFITS Relaxes muscles; slows heart and breathing rate; calms the nervous system; improves sleep quality by soothing and clearing the mind.

TIME Around 4 minutes. Ideally practise every night before bed.

ITEMS NEEDED Yoga mat or towel.

PREPARATION Ensure the room is warm. Wear loose, comfortable clothing.

02

Rolling like a ball Take your legs down from the wall and hug your knees to your chest, clasping your hands around your shins. Inhale and rock to a sitting position, then exhale as you roll back down. Roll up and down in this way for up to 1 minute.

03

Corpse Release your clasped hands and lower your knees to lie flat on your back, legs straight. Put your arms down by your sides, palms facing upwards. Relax and rest here for up to 1 minute.

In rolling like a ball, knees should be as close to your head as feels comfortable

Curve your back to help you as you rock

01

Warm a little oil between your hands. Use your palms to make small, back and forth motions all over your scalp for 2 minutes.

02

For the foot massage, cross your right ankle over your left knee. Take more oil and use your left palm to rub the top of your right foot from ankle to toes.

BEDTIME SCALP AND FOOT MASSAGE

In Ayurveda many *srotamsi* (the channels through which life energy flows) begin in the scalp and end in the soles of our feet. In this massage, you unblock these channels and prepare yourself for sleep by releasing any impurities and negative energies that have accumulated during the day.

04

Now repeat steps 2 and 3 for your left foot, using more oil if needed. Put on a pair of socks to help your feet retain the nourishing properties of the oil while you sleep.

03

Now rub the back of your right foot from ankle to heel. Then, using the thumbs of both hands, massage the sole of your right foot.

NEED TO KNOW

BENEFITS Moisturizes the skin; reduces tension and stress by clearing mental blockages; releases trapped emotions.

TIME Around 6 minutes: 2 minutes for scalp massage, around 2 minutes for each foot massage. Ideally perform nightly just before going to bed.

ITEMS NEEDED 2–3 tsp cured sesame oil; socks to wear overnight.

HEALING
PRACTICES

These simple practices – including herbal preparations, medicinal foods, and massage routines – can be tailored to your individual needs to help you to identify, relieve, manage, and prevent specific causes of ill health, and restore balance to your entire being.

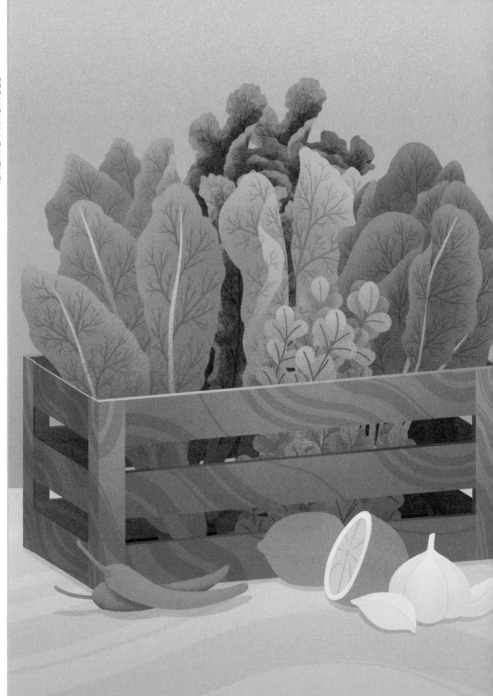

CHOLESTEROL-BALANCING GREENS

In Ayurveda, high cholesterol is caused by excess kapha dosha, and a disturbance of *meda dhatu*, the fat tissue. Balancing kapha and keeping *meda dhatu* healthy is the key to keeping cholesterol in check.

Cholesterol – fat made in the liver – is essential for our bodies to function properly, but too much will clog the arteries. High cholesterol is often caused by an overly fatty diet and excess kapha dosha. Following the principles of Ayurvedic nutrition (see pages 22–23) will keep kapha dosha in check, as will taking regular exercise, to counteract kapha's static and dense qualities with vata's movement.

SAUTÉED GREENS

Including plenty of bitter greens in your diet will cut through kapha's heavy, sticky, and oily qualities. Dress cooked greens with salt and lime juice – the sharpness and acidity will further reduce kapha. This makes a delicious, kapha-reducing side accompaniment to any meal:

Ingredients – serves 1
• 2 large handfuls of a mixture of shredded greens such as kale, mustard leaves, spinach, chard, and fenugreek leaves
• 1 garlic clove, thinly sliced
• 1 small red chilli, finely sliced
• 1½ tsp in total of equal parts fenugreek, fennel, cumin, coriander, and mustard seeds
• ½ tsp turmeric powder
• 1 tsp organic ghee
• Pinch of rock salt
• Squeeze of lime juice

Fry the garlic in the ghee for a few seconds, then add the chilli and spices, before throwing in the greens. Mix well and sauté for a few minutes. Tip the greens onto a serving plate and top with the salt and lime.

TREATING SPOTS
AND ACNE

In Ayurveda, spots and acne are often a sign of pitta dosha and *rakta* (blood) problems. The key to managing these often-distressing conditions is to tame fiery pitta and clear the blood of toxins.

When excess pitta circulates in the bloodstream and accumulates in the outer layer of the skin, it can cause spots, soreness, and redness. In mainstream medicine, people with acne are often given oral and topical antibiotics, or steroid skin creams. When taken for long periods, antibiotics can upset the delicate balance of our natural gut bacteria, and steroids weaken the skin's structure.

While it's important to seek medical advice if your acne is severe, Ayurvedic treatments, which focus on lowering pitta dosha and detoxifying the blood, can be very effective for milder cases of acne and occasional breakouts.

Purify the blood Proper digestion is key to keeping the blood clear of toxins. Eat calming, pitta-reducing foods such as asparagus, cucumber, and leafy greens. Drinking warm water flavoured with a good squeeze of lime juice will also help to purify the blood, as limes are high in antioxidants.

Manage dairy intake Dairy can be eaten in moderation, but must not be

"A cooling herbal paste can be applied to the skin to treat spots and acne effectively."

mixed with incompatible foods. Never eat dairy with fruit or fish, as this increases pitta. Avoid hard cheese as it is tamasic – *tamas* is the energy of heaviness and lethargy, which can lead to improper digestion, causing further outbreaks.

De-stress yourself Stress also represents an excess of pitta dosha, so can trigger or worsen spots and acne. For an effective stress management technique, see pages 60–61.

Healing paste This treatment is made from wonderfully cooling sandalwood, turmeric, and rosewater, and will calm inflammation. Mix half a teaspoon of sandalwood powder and a pinch of turmeric powder with half a teaspoon of gram (chickpea) flour. Add a few drops of rosewater and stir to form a smooth paste. Apply to affected areas of the skin, and leave for 10 minutes. Rinse off gently, and pat your skin dry with a clean towel. Use a cotton-wool pad soaked in rosewater to remove any residue.

REHYDRATING DRY, ITCHY SKIN

In Ayurveda, itchy, flaky skin irritations, and in particular eczema, are caused by an imbalance in all three doshas. Treatment focuses on soothing the symptoms, and on restoring balance to prevent future outbreaks.

When food is not digested properly, ama forms and circulate around the body. Pitta dosha's warmth can heat these toxins, which aggravates the skin. Itchiness can also be triggered by too much vata dosha dryness, and also insufficient kapha, leading the skin to become brittle from a lack of natural oils and moisture. Follow the Ayurvedic routine (pages 26–27) to ensure proper digestion and balance in the three doshas.

PLANT MEDICINES

The neem tree is a flowering tree from India; neem oil is extracted from the seeds of its fruit. Neem oil is antiseptic, antibacterial, antiviral, and anti-inflammatory and soothes skin irritations, especially eczema.

Massage neem oil gently over affected areas of the body every day after bathing.

Aloe vera is cooling, and anti-inflammatory. The gel found inside its leaves is intensely moisturizing, and penetrates the skin quickly and deeply to counteract vata's dryness and promote healing. If you have an aloe vera plant at home, pinch a leaf between your fingers and gently pull it off from where it joins the stem. Take a knife, carefully slit the leaf, and scrape out the gel inside. Rub this into itchy skin after bathing; unused gel can be stored in the fridge for up to 10 days. You can also buy aloe vera gel from any good pharmacy or health shop.

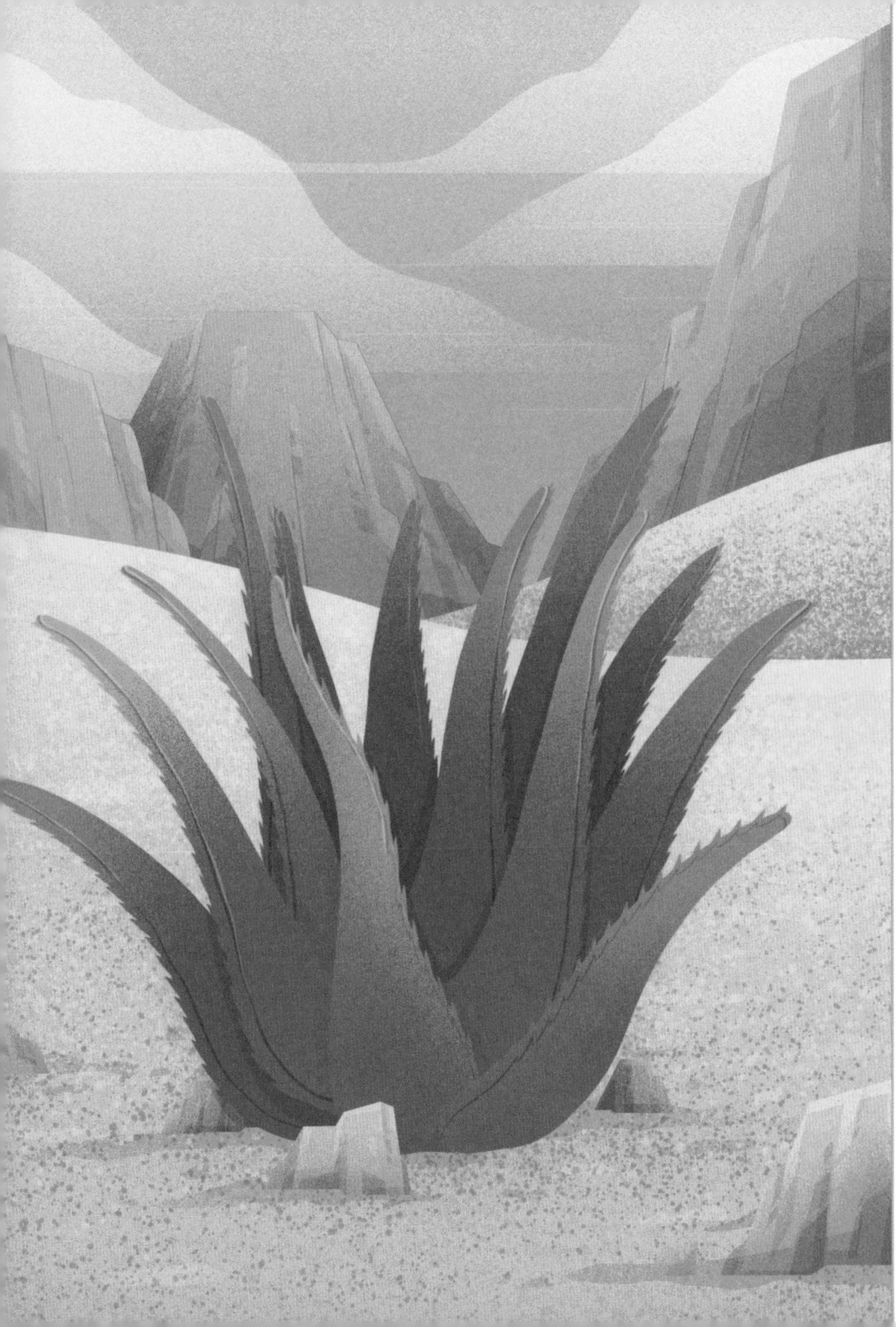

REFRESH DRY, STRAINED, AND TIRED EYES

With ever-increasing use of computers and other digital devices, our eyes take a great deal of daily strain. Try these Ayurvedic techniques to rejuvenate overworked eyes.

Many eye problems arise from an excess of pitta dosha. Feeling stressed, angry, or anxious can put additional strain on our eyes, as can alcohol, spicy food, direct sunlight, and pollution as these all contain pitta's hot quality, which dries out the eyes. Ayurvedic remedies focus on restoring balance to the doshas, but be sure to seek professional advice if your eyesight suddenly worsens, or for any eye injuries.

PITTA-REDUCING TECHNIQUES

Tired eyes Massaging your scalp and feet (see pages 98–99) is a great way to cool the heat of pitta, and draw it away from your eyes. By unblocking your energy channels, you allow excess pitta dosha to flow from your body.

Eye strain If your vision has started to blur, rosewater will not only temper pitta's heat, but it is also wonderfully nourishing for the tissues of your eyelids, helping to revive them. Soak two cotton-wool pads in organic, pure rosewater that has been cooled in the fridge, then squeeze excess rosewater out of the pads. Lie down, close your eyes, and place a pad over each eye for 10 minutes.

Dry eyes If your eyes sting or feel sensitive, use a sterile dropper to put a drop of liquified, lukewarm, organic ghee in each eye just before you go to sleep. The high, pure fat content in ghee will restore the moisture that pitta's heat has dried out.

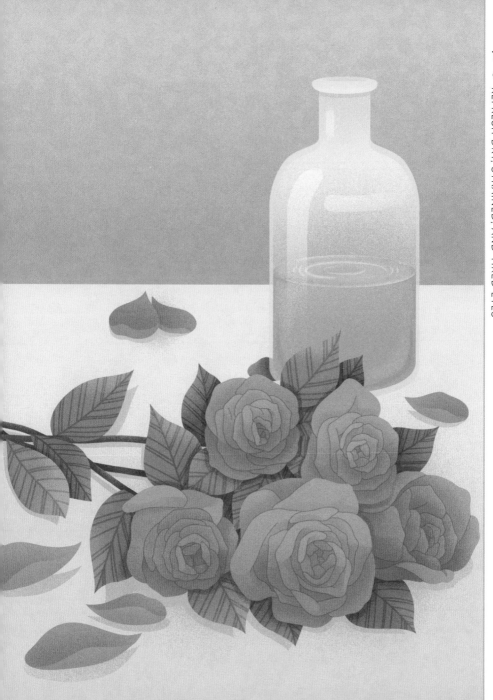

MANAGING MENSTRUATION

Most women experience physical and emotional changes at different points in their menstrual cycle. According to Ayurveda, uncomfortable symptoms are due to an imbalance in the doshas, and can be alleviated by targeting the dosha responsible for each problem.

Menstruation has different stages, each dominated by a particular dosha. First is vata dosha, moving the blood downwards and out of the body during the 3–7 days of your period. The second stage, at the end of bleeding, is the kapha phase. Ovulation occurs around day 14 of a woman's cycle at the cusp of the kapha and pitta phases – pitta being the phase after ovulation leading up to your next period. Ayurveda can help you to manage the symptoms that accompany each stage by targeting the dosha affected.

VATA MANAGEMENT

Issues caused by vata imbalances during the time of your period include anxiety, fear, mood swings, and feeling distracted. Try this vata-soothing milk drink each night before you go to bed during this stage of your cycle: add a generous pinch of ground ginger and nutmeg to 200ml of milk and bring to the boil. Pour into a mug and add a half-teaspoon of ghee. The heat of the ginger and lubrication from the ghee will counteract vata's cool movement, and nutmeg aids sleep.

"Symptoms can be managed by adding the opposite qualities of the dosha causing the problem."

KAPHA MANAGEMENT

In the pre-ovulation stage, kapha symptoms can include bloating, puffiness, feeling heavy or sluggish, a low mood, and excess sleepiness. *Abhyanga* (a self-massage with warm oil) can be very helpful in managing kapha symptoms – see pages 44–45 for steps. Add half a teaspoon of Himalayan rock salt to your massage oil – this will stimulate your skin and reach the deep tissues, which will ease stagnation and help movement in the body.

PITTA MANAGEMENT

Pitta symptoms include anger or irritation, an increase in body temperature, and tender breasts. Drink warm, previously boiled water, and add plenty of fresh mint leaves which are balancing for all three doshas. Sip throughout the day. For tender breasts, temper pitta's fire by gently massaging them for 5 minutes each day using 1 teaspoon of cured sesame oil with 2 drops of cooling rose essential oil added.

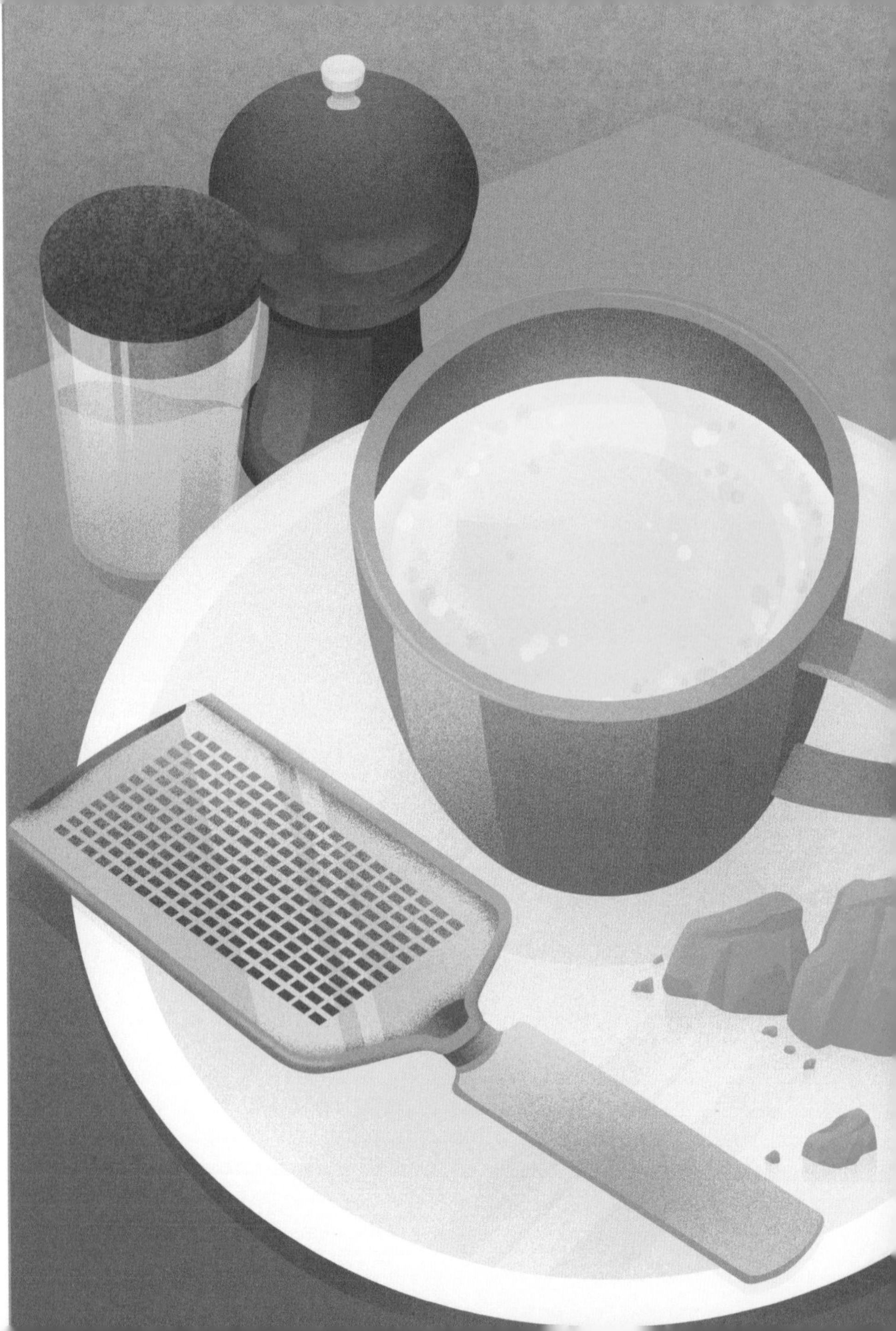

TRADITIONAL TURMERIC COUGH AND COLD REMEDY

This easy-to-make drink is a traditional Ayurvedic remedy known as *haldi doodh* (turmeric milk) that boosts immunity, clears the airways, and soothes the throat. It can relieve coughs and colds, as well as prevent them. The powerful healing properties of the turmeric are balancing for all doshas – creating peace and harmony in the mind and body.

NEED TO KNOW:

BENEFITS Dries out excess mucus; soothes and clears airways; anti-inflammatory and antiseptic properties.

TIME Around 5 minutes to prepare.

To treat symptoms, drink before bedtime to ensure a better night's sleep.

To prevent seasonal coughs and colds, drink 3 times a week during winter.

INGREDIENTS
Makes 1 serving

- 280ml whole milk (or non-dairy milk)
- ¼ tsp turmeric powder
- ¼ tsp ground black pepper
- Grated jaggery or raw honey

01

Add the milk, turmeric, and black pepper to a small saucepan and stir well.

02

Gently warm on a medium heat until the milk just begins to boil, then immediately take off the heat.

03

Allow to cool a little, then add a small amount of grated jaggery or raw honey to sweeten. Stir well and pour into a mug. Drink while still warm.

REDUCING YOUR RISK OF DIABETES

If you've been told you are at risk of developing Type 2 diabetes, an Ayurvedic routine can help you address your diet and lifestyle. An excess of kapha dosha is indicated in this condition, so decreasing this is key to reducing risk.

In Type 2 diabetes, the body has become resistant to insulin, a hormone that controls blood sugar levels. If your blood sugar level is higher than it should be, this can be a warning sign. Your doctor may tell you that you are pre-diabetic, or at higher risk of developing diabetes. Type 2 diabetes can be partly genetic, but is heavily influenced by diet and lifestyle, so making healthy choices in these areas can help to reduce your risk of developing this disease.

According to Ayurveda, excess kapha dosha and *meda dhatu* (fat tissue) are both involved in the onset of Type 2 diabetes. Kapha is cold, slow, heavy, static, soft, and oily. When a person has excess kapha, they also tend to display all these qualities, having both a heaviness in their body and mind, and excessively moist or oily skin.

If you have already been diagnosed diabetic, an Ayurvedic routine can help you manage the condition, but you will also need to follow the medical advice of your doctor.

" Fenugreek seeds can help to slow digestion and balance blood sugar levels naturally."

Nutrition Avoid heavy or sugary foods such as red meat, cheese, biscuits and cakes, fizzy drinks and alcohol, which are rich in kapha. These foods are poorly digested, leading to a build-up of toxins, and contributing to the development of unhealthy, fatty tissues. Instead, include lots of complex carbohydrates such as brown rice, wholewheat pasta, and quinoa, which all pacify kapha.

Exercise Physical activity has the vata qualities of lightness and movement, which help to stimulate metabolism and counteract kapha. Exercising every day, even just a brisk walk for 20 minutes, will help to keep kapha in check.

Herbal drink Fenugreek lowers blood sugar naturally by regulating how our body absorbs carbohydrates and sugars. Every morning, add 2 teaspoons of fenugreek seeds to 300ml of water and boil for 5–10 minutes until the liquid has turned green, and has reduced by a third in volume. Strain to remove the seeds, and allow to cool slightly before drinking on an empty stomach.

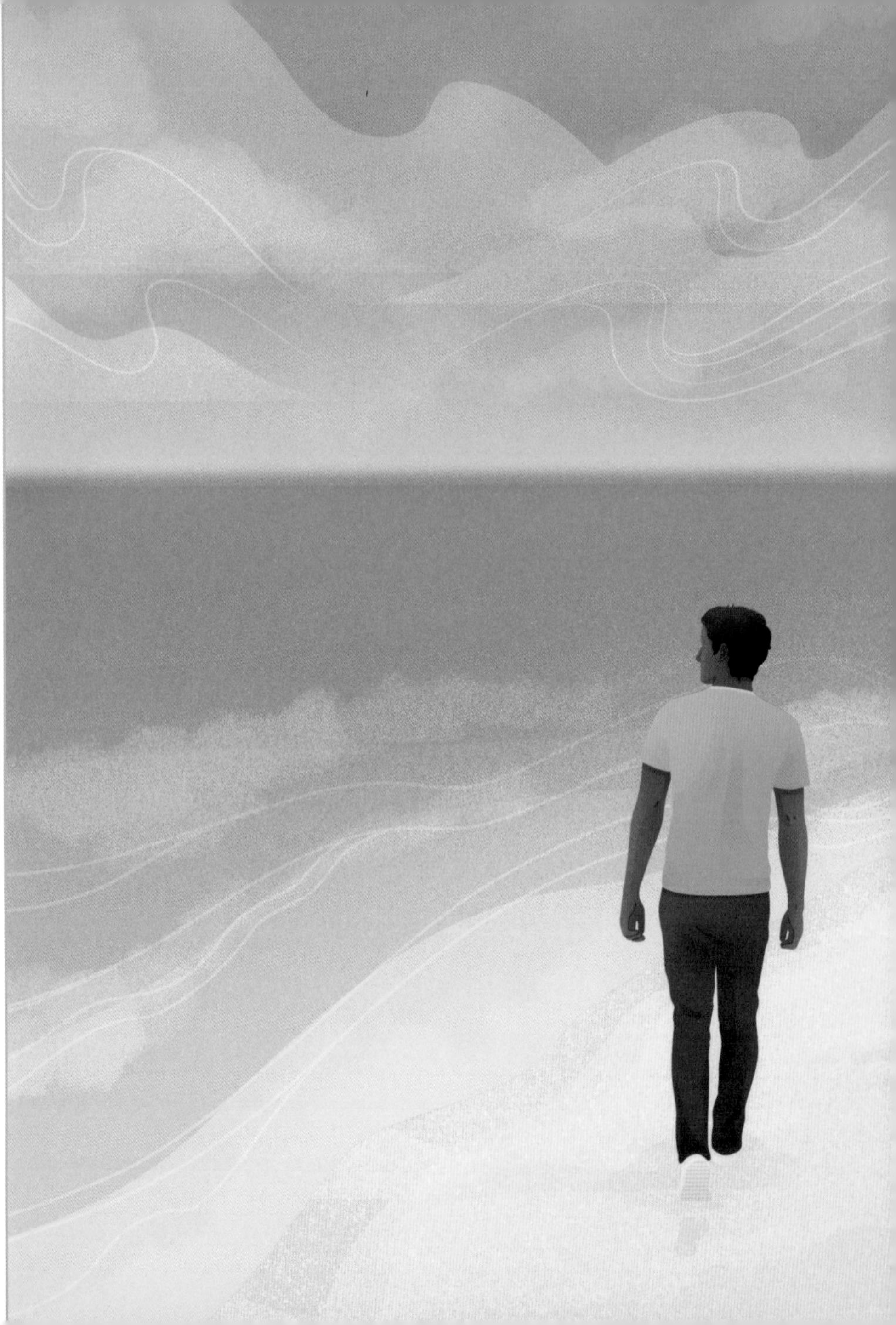

OVERCOME BREATHING PROBLEMS

Some breathing disorders can be the result of too much kapha. Soothe symptoms with kapha-balancing foods, an active lifestyle, and an ancient Ayurvedic spice remedy.

Coughing, breathlessness and wheezing are some of the unpleasant, and at times distressing, symptoms of asthma and other respiratory conditions. These are triggered by too much kapha dosha, which causes the lungs to overproduce mucus, leading to dampness, stickiness, and heaviness. Excess kapha can be a result of lifestyle issues, or outside factors such as air pollution and allergens.

Balance kapha Restrict foods that are very sweet, sour, salty, heavy, and oily. These all have kapha qualities, which will trigger further mucus production. Instead, choose foods and spices that are bitter, pungent, and astringent such as garlic, ginger, turmeric, coriander, and chillies which dry up the excess liquid of kapha. Regular exercise, such as walking or yoga, will add vata's movement, which counteracts kapha's stickiness.

Spice remedy *Trikatu*, Sanskrit for "three pungents", is an ancient Ayurvedic remedy for respiratory issues. Mix together equal parts of dry ginger powder, ground black pepper, and long pepper powder, and store them in a screw-top jar. Mix a pinch of this *trikatu* mixture, plus a pinch of turmeric, with half a teaspoon of raw honey and take twice a day, followed by a sip of warm water. The pungent spices strip the lung tissues and cells of fatty kapha deposits, helping to restore balance and allowing you to breathe more easily.

MANAGE THE MENOPAUSE

For women, menopause is a time of transition from the pitta to vata stage of life, and can bring challenging symptoms. Manage them successfully by keeping pitta and vata dosha in balance.

Symptoms of menopause can vary from woman to woman and range from the mood swings and hot flushes caused by the excess heat of pitta dosha, to headaches and insomnia caused by the drying effects of vata dosha imbalances. Ayurvedic remedies can soothe symptoms by enabling the doshas to regain balance.

MANAGE VATA

Counteract vata's dryness by eating stewed fruits rather than raw, which are easier to digest; and unsalted nuts and seeds, which are rich in natural oils. **Fenugreek** has properties that can help reduce the symptoms of menopause: it is most effective when taken as a herbal tea infusion. Add a tablespoon of fenugreek seeds to 1 litre of water and heat gently in a pan on a medium heat for 5–10 minutes. Once brewed, strain the tea through a sieve to remove the seeds, then pour into a vacuum flask to keep warm. Sip regularly throughout the day.

"*Cooling asparagus helps to balance the heat of pitta, which can cause hot flushes and irritability.*"

MANAGE PITTA

To soothe the heat of pitta, eat cooling greens and avoid chillies, salt, and alcohol – these can worsen symptoms. **Asparagus** is used in Ayurveda for hormonal balance. It is also an anti-inflammatory and antioxidant, and so excellent for reducing excess pitta dosha. A tasty way to eat asparagus is as a soup. Heat 2 teaspoons of ghee and 1 teaspoon of oil in a pan. Add a small, finely chopped onion and fry until soft. Add a large clove of finely chopped garlic, 250g of fresh, chopped asparagus, and 50g of peeled, chopped potatoes. Cook for 5 minutes, then add ¼ teaspoon of turmeric powder and ½ a teaspoon each of ground coriander and cumin. Stir well, then add 300ml of vegetable stock. Bring to the boil for 1 minute, then cover and reduce the heat to simmer for 10–15 minutes. Once cool, blend, return to the pan to warm gently, then serve.

01

Sit comfortably on a chair with your back straight and feet firmly on the floor. Relax your shoulders and place your hands, palms facing upwards, in your lap.

02

Close your eyes and soften your mouth, so it is slightly open. Observe your breathing, and allow it to come to a slow, steady rhythm.

POSITIVE AFFIRMATION

It can be easy to become preoccupied with our shortcomings and worry about how others see us, but this can steer us away from our true selves. This ritual, which involves reciting a positive statement about yourself, will help you embrace the truth that you are good enough.

04

Take a few more deep, soothing breaths before opening your eyes and turning your mind to your goals for the day.

03

Silently repeat the following positive affirmation to yourself for at least five minutes: "I lovingly nourish my unique mind, body, and spirit with only what it needs. I know what is good for my holistic health. That alone is all I need."

NEED TO KNOW

BENEFITS Steers you away from negative thoughts and self-doubt; helps to identify true goals; improves focus; brings inner peace and clarity; balances the doshas.

TIME Around 5 minutes. Perform if you start to find yourself obsessing over making decisions, or feel low in self-esteem.

KEEP ANXIETY AT BAY

Anxiety results from a vata dosha disturbance. Vata is light, mobile, and airy, and if these qualities become excessive, they can agitate the nervous system. Managing this condition focuses on restoring balance to, and grounding, vata.

If you live with anxiety you may struggle to control your worries, feel tired or irritable, find it difficult to concentrate, and suffer poor or disrupted sleep. If you are already a vata-dominant person and your nutrition and lifestyle choices lead to a further increase of this dosha, you may find you are more prone to suffering from anxiety. Being extra mindful of your routines and anything that adds excess vata is important.

BALANCING VATA

Yoga The practice of yoga is very effective for calming the mind. Even if you only manage 5–10 minutes of every day, you will feel the benefits. Both mountain and corpse pose (see pages 34–35 and 96–97) are particularly stabilizing, bringing flighty vata back down to earth.

Walk barefoot Walking barefoot outdoors (when the weather allows) will help you to absorb the grounding

" Keeping vata dosha in check will reduce the likelihood of you suffering from anxiety."

properties of the earth, taking in its solid kapha qualities and bringing stability to an anxious, restless mind.

Tulsi tea remedy The tulsi plant, known as "holy basil", is highly revered in Ayurveda as it is adaptogenic, which means it helps the body adapt to stressors. Tulsi is also a natural antidepressant, its heating qualities helping to balance out excess vata dosha. Known to many as "the elixir of life", tulsi promotes an overall sense of wellbeing. To make tulsi tea, take 8–10 whole tulsi leaves and infuse them in 600ml of hot water. Keeping the leaves, pour the tea into a vacuum flask and sip throughout the day to benefit from its soothing effects. You can grow your own tulsi plant at home – plants are available to buy at garden centres or nurseries. Alternatively you can buy tulsi leaves from wholefood or Indian food shops.

RELIEVING HEADACHES

We all suffer headaches from time to time. In Ayurveda, headaches are described as vata, pitta, or kapha types, depending on how the pain feels. They are often a signal that we need to bring balance to the doshas.

Headaches can be caused by a variety of factors, such as stress or illness. Treating the root cause is the best long-term solution, but you can manage your symptoms Ayurvedically in the short term. If you have persistent or frequent headaches, see your doctor.

Vata headaches cause a dull, throbbing sensation and are usually triggered by day-to-day stress. To treat these, drink warm water with a little grated ginger root – the heat counteracts vata's cold. Grounding and nourishing sesame oil can also be used to calm vata's mobility and dryness. Tip your head right back and put three drops of warmed oil into each nostril.

Pitta headaches can produce a sharp, intense burning, as well as nausea and light-sensitivity. To temper pitta's fire, boil water with a teaspoon of sweet, cool fennel seeds. Strain to remove seeds and drink at room temperature. You can also soothe the heat of this type of headache by melting a little cooling coconut oil between your palms or in a pan, then massaging into the scalp.

Kapha headaches tend to make you feel foggy and lethargic. They are usually caused by sinus congestion, colds, and allergies, or too much sleep. Drink water that has been boiled with the seeds of two light, sweet cardamoms to counteract kapha's density. You can also cut through kapha's heaviness by inhaling steam infused with head-clearing eucalyptus oil.

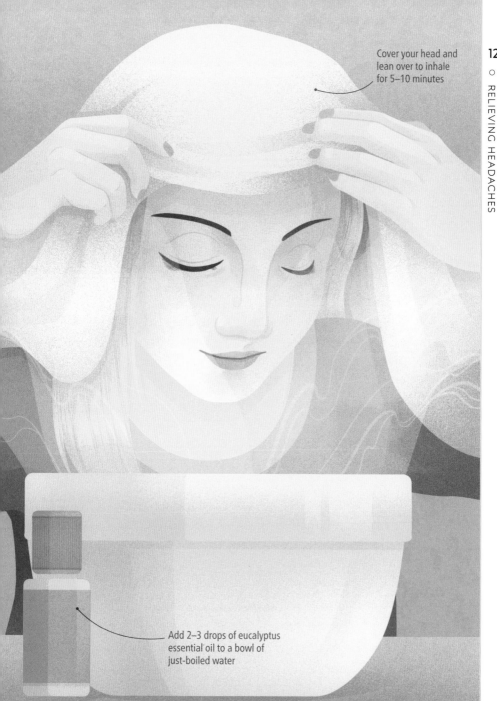

Cover your head and lean over to inhale for 5–10 minutes

Add 2–3 drops of eucalyptus essential oil to a bowl of just-boiled water

DIARRHOEA AND CONSTIPATION

When food isn't properly digested and absorbed by
your body, diarrhoea or constipation can be the result.
Balancing pitta and vata doshas will bring welcome relief
from these unpleasant conditions.

DIARRHOEA

If your stools are loose and watery, it may
be your body's way of trying to flush toxins,
contaminated food, or even medications
from your system too quickly. In Ayurveda,
diarrhoea and its associated discomfort
is linked to excess pitta dosha and
weakened agni, so it's important to
address both to rebalance your system.

During a bout of diarrhoea, drink plenty
of room-temperature water to ensure
your body stays hydrated and stick to
bland foods, such as the following recipe.

If diarrhoea lasts more than three days,
seek your doctor's advice.

Rice and yoghurt remedy Basmati rice
helps to bind stools, balances all three
doshas, is highly nourishing, and
easy for agni to digest. Plain yoghurt
contains healthy bacteria to replace the
essential gut microbes that can be lost
with diarrhoea. Mix together 125g of
freshly cooked basmati rice, 30g of plain,
organic yoghurt, and 2 teaspoons organic
ghee (see pages 48–49). Eat slowly, and
sip room-temperature water as you do so.

"*Over— or understimulation of the bowels occurs when pitta and vata doshas are out of balance.*"

CONSTIPATION

With constipation, you struggle to have bowel movements, or to fully empty your bowels. You might sense a heaviness in your intestines. The cold, hard, dry qualities of vata dosha are associated with constipation – you may have been eating too many cold or drying foods, or not drinking enough water. If you have been feeling afraid or lonely, these vata emotions can also trigger symptoms. To relieve constipation, choose food and drink that stimulates agni, such as this tea recipe below. If constipation lasts more than two weeks, see your doctor.

Cumin, coriander, and fennel tea
Renowned for their bowel-stimulating abilities, these spices support the downward movement of vata dosha. Add a teaspoon each of cumin, fennel, and coriander seeds to a litre of water and simmer for 15 minutes. Strain through a sieve to remove the seeds and store in a vacuum flask to keep warm. Sip throughout the day.

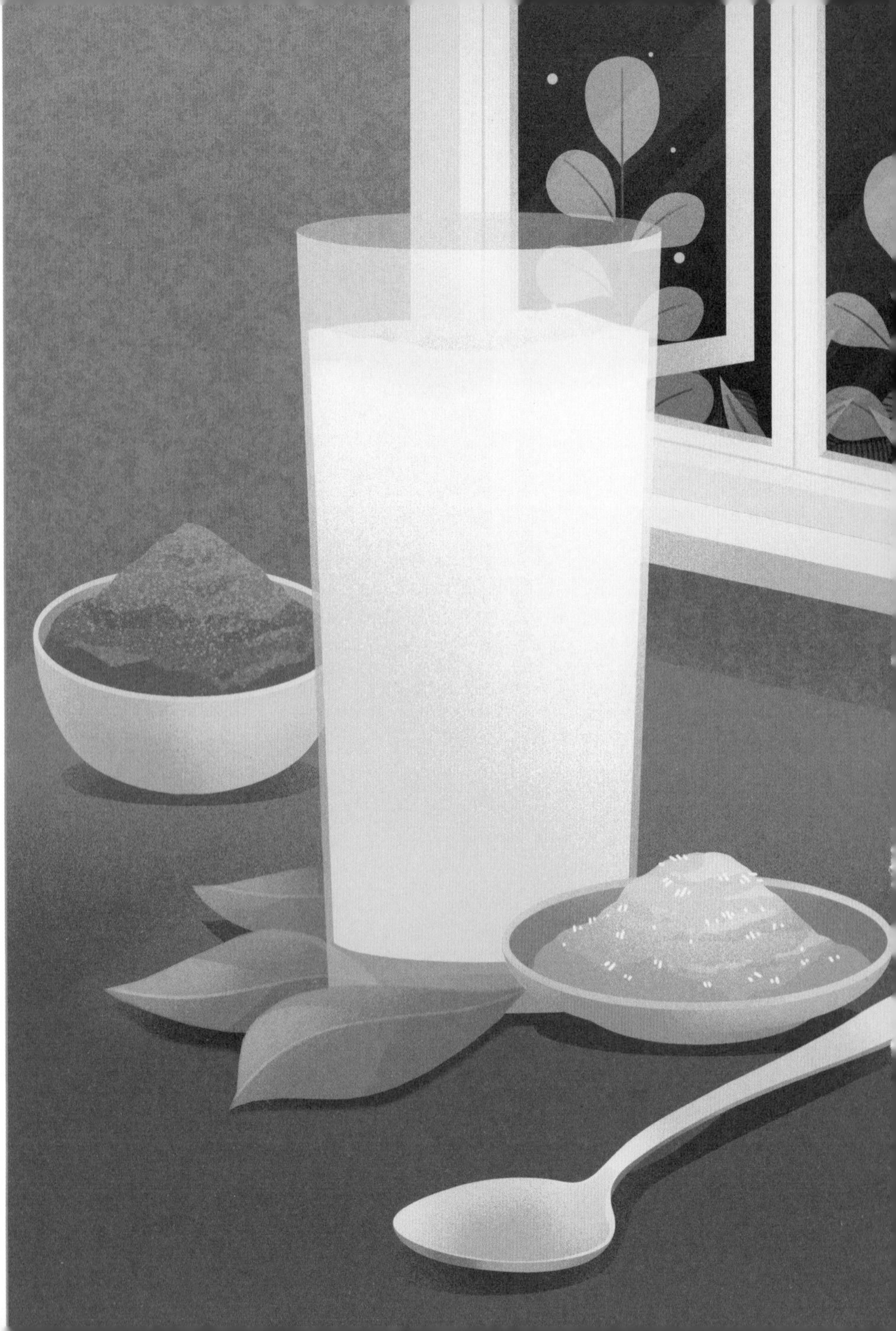

LASSI DRINK TO SOOTHE HEARTBURN

Lassi is a traditional Indian drink made from yoghurt, water, and spices, which helps relieve the discomfort of heartburn and indigestion. Drink a glass of lassi after eating to help agni break down food and counteract the burning heat of pitta dosha.

NEED TO KNOW

BENEFITS Reduces excess stomach acid; cooling and digestive properties reduce pitta dosha; contains beneficial bacteria which speed the digestive process; particularly good for the frequent heartburn experienced during pregnancy.

TIME 3 minutes to prepare. Drink daily after lunch and evening meals as needed.

INGREDIENTS
Makes 2 glasses

- 150ml whole-milk yoghurt
- 300ml cold water
- ¼ teaspoon ground cumin
- ¼ teaspoon Himalayan rock salt
- 12 fresh curry leaves

CAUTION If indigestion or heartburn last for more than 3 weeks, see your doctor.

01

Place the yoghurt and water in a blender. Add the ground cumin and salt. Blend on a low pulse setting for 30 seconds.

02

Add the curry leaves to the mixture and blend for another 15 seconds, until smooth and frothy. Pour the lassi into glasses to serve.

03

Sip the lassi slowly at the end of your meal. When you have finished the drink, sit quietly for at least 5 minutes to allow agni time and space to start its work on digesting your food.

01

Lie on your back on a bed, with knees bent and feet flat on the bed's surface. Lightly coat your hands with the oil. Breathe slowly and deeply.

02

Begin on your right side, at your pelvic bone. Use your palms and fingers to make small, circular motions over your abdomen, working upwards to your rib cage.

SOOTHING ABDOMINAL MASSAGE FOR IBS

In Ayurveda, undigested food or suppressed emotions can disrupt agni and lead to irritable bowel syndrome (IBS). This comforting massage helps to ease symptoms such as bloating, abdominal cramps, and fatigue by supporting agni and improving the flow of digestive juices into the gut.

03

Now massage just under your rib cage, moving across to your left side, then massage all the way down your left side to the pelvic bone.

05

Taking more oil if you need to, repeat steps 2–4 until your symptoms ease. To finish, wipe off any excess oil and lie quietly for a few minutes before you get up.

04

Bring both hands to your navel and use your fingertips to make small clockwise circles, pressing a little deeper if this is comfortable.

NEED TO KNOW

BENEFITS Relieves pain and cramps; supports vata dosha by promoting movement of food downwards through the intestines; relaxes muscles and relieves excess gas.

TIME Around 5–10 minutes. Perform as often as needed, when uncomfortable symptoms begin.

ITEMS NEEDED 1–2 tsp cured sesame oil; towel.

CAUTION If you think you may have IBS, see a doctor.

EASE BACK PAIN

In Ayurveda, problems with bones and the skeleton are associated with too much of vata dosha's light, mobile, and brittle qualities. Pain is also a vata function, so treating back pain focuses on decreasing excess vata dosha.

Vata's cold, dry, hard, and rough qualities can all contribute to back pain. Vata can especially creep in when you are in cold conditions for long periods of time. In Ayurveda, emotions always play a key role: the spine needs stability, so if you feel unsupported emotionally, you may also experience back pain. Here are a few ways in which an Ayurvedic approach can ease the misery of back pain: however, if discomfort does not improve after three weeks, you should see your doctor.

TARGETING THE CAUSES

Use a support in your lower back area, and around your shoulders, to prevent slouching when you are sitting for long spells. This offers the spine the stability it needs, counteracting vata's mobility. **Yoga** keeps the back supple and free of tension, as well as increasing blood flow, which will warm the body and counteract vata's cold and dry properties. See pages 34–35, 82–83 and 96–97 for some simple postures to try.

> " *The heat of pitta will reduce dry, mobile vata and relieve your back pain.* "

Journaling (see pages 66–67) is a way of processing your experiences and emotions through writing them down. It can help you stabilize any thoughts and feelings that are adding to your back pain.

GARLIC OIL MASSAGE

A massage with warm garlic oil is a great way to counteract vata's cold, dry properties. The friction from rubbing creates warmth, and the garlic has pitta dosha qualities that also temper vata.

In a pan, gently warm 2 tablespoons of castor oil and a peeled clove of garlic for about 5 minutes. Remove the garlic and let the oil cool slightly before gently rubbing it into your lower back in smooth, circular strokes. Continue for around 10 minutes, or until tension eases. If possible, massage after bathing when your skin is still warm and slightly damp – the oil will lock in the moisture. If you have a willing helper, lie on your stomach and have them massage the painful areas for you.

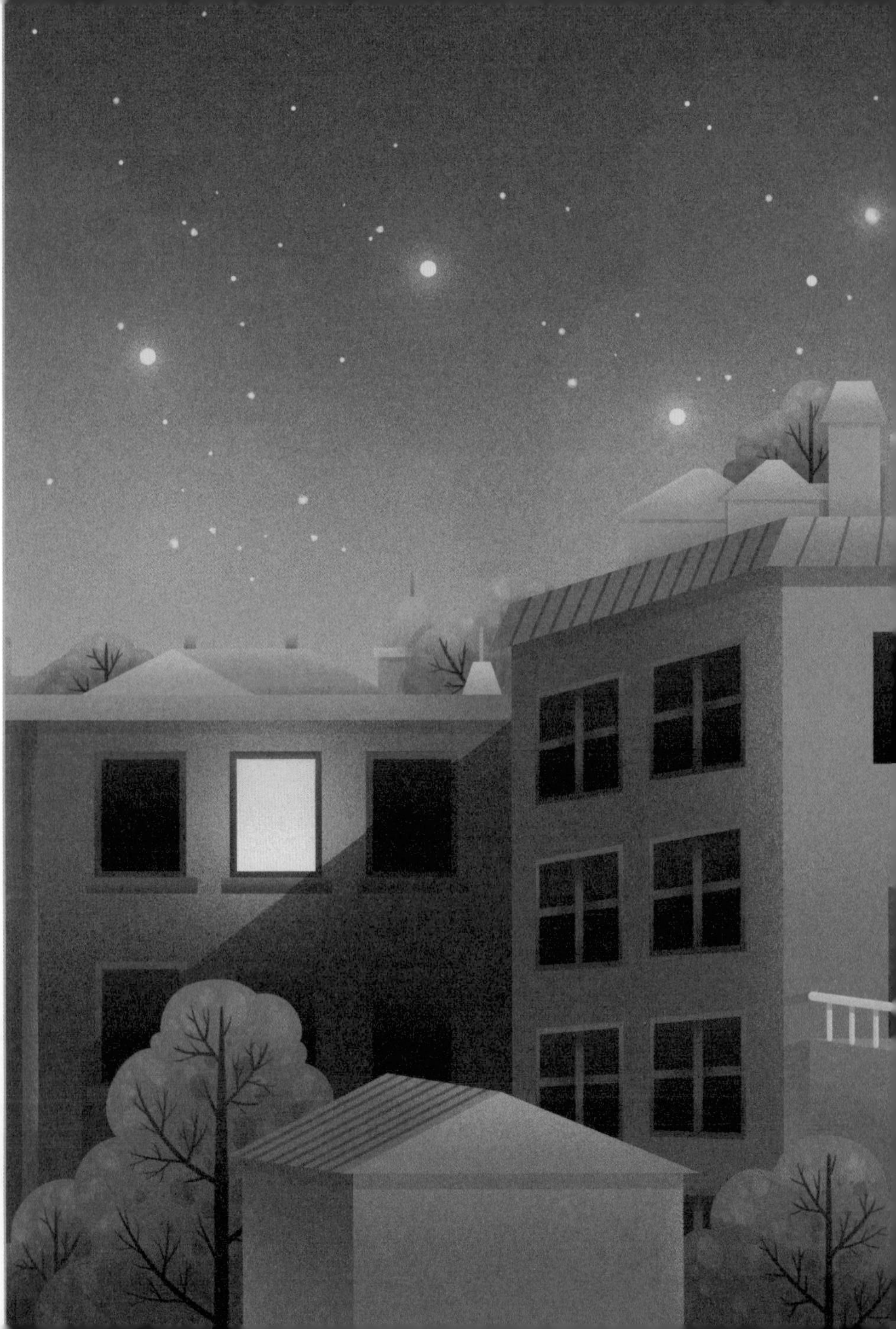

BEATING INSOMNIA

Sleep is essential for both health and happiness – a precious time to restore and replenish the body and mind. If you have sleep problems, an Ayurvedic approach can often help you get the rest you need.

Insomnia is associated with an excess of vata and pitta doshas. Both have lightness, mobility and ungroundedness, whereas sleep requires kapha's static quality as well as its heaviness and stability. Our busy lives create a hostile environment for sleep: hectic work schedules, irregular routines, late nights, working on screens, and day-to-day worries all cause excess vata and pitta, keeping our minds active when we should be sleeping.

Use your bedroom only for sleep – working, watching TV, or eating in your bedroom all encourage the lively, fast-moving properties of pitta and vata to enter your sleeping space.

Switch off digital devices after your evening meal. The light from these devices disrupts your internal clock, keeping your body on high alert, instead of letting it prepare for rest. **Avoid alcohol and caffeine** in the evening; both are stimulants and increase pitta dosha's sharpness. **Take a warm bath** with 5 drops of lavender essential oil (see pages 52–53) an hour before bed. Lavender has kapha's calming properties. **Have a milky drink** half an hour before bed. Add a pinch of nutmeg and a ¼ teaspoon of ghee to a mug of hot milk. Nutmeg is sleep-enhancing, while ghee helps to replenish the body's tissues.

RESOURCES

These pages offer some recommended reading, information, and resources to further your Ayurvedic knowledge and practice. If you would like professional support, or if you require treatment for more complex or long-term conditions, see the directories section for help finding a qualified Ayurvedic Medicine Practitioner.

FURTHER READING

Practical Ayurveda Sivananda Yoga Vedanta Centre (DK)

Textbook of Ayurveda: Volume 1: Fundamental Principles Vasant Lad (Ayurvedic Press)

Ayurveda and the Mind Dr David Frawley (Lotus Press)

The Complete Book of Ayurvedic Home Remedies Vasant Lad (Harmony)

Ayurveda: A Life of Balance Maya Tiwari (Motilal Banarsidass)

Ayurveda (Idiot's Guides) Sahara Rose Ketabi (Alpha)

ONLINE RESOURCES

The Ayurvedic Institute
www.ayurveda.com

The Chopra Center
www.chopra.com

Banyan Botanicals
www.banyanbotanicals.com

Essential Ayurveda
www.essentialayurveda.co.uk

RELATED READING

B.K.S. Iyengar Yoga: The Path to Holistic Health B.K.S. Iyengar (DK)

The Complete Illustrated Guide to Aromatherapy Julia Lawless (Element Books)

The Vision: Reflections on the Way of the Soul Kahlil Gibran (Penguin)

The Alchemist Paulo Coelho (HarperCollins)

PRACTITIONER DIRECTORIES/ASSOCIATIONS

Ayurvedic Professionals Association (APA)
www.apa.uk.com

Association of Ayurvedic Professionals UK (AAPUK)
www.aapuk.net

The British Association of Accredited Ayurvedic Practitioners (BAAAP)
www.britayurpractitioners.com

The British Wheel of Yoga
www.bwy.org.uk

International Ayurveda Congress
www.internationalayurvedacongress.com

European Ayurveda Association
www.euroayurveda.eu

PRIVATE SESSIONS AND TRAINING

Private consultations with personalized health and wellbeing
programmes, as well as ongoing Ayurvedic holistic health
support are available with Sonja Shah-Williams. Sonja also
offers mentoring and training sessions for practitioners by appointment.

For more information contact:
Sonja Shah-Williams
www.anala.co.uk

GLOSSARY

ABHYANGA
Self-massage with warm oil; a key
component of Ayurvedic healing practices.

AGNI
The digestive fire. Agni needs to be kept
in peak condition to digest our food
properly, create healthy dhatus (tissues),
and produce ojas (immunity).

AMA
Toxins created by undigested food and
unprocessed emotions. If these build up
they will begin to circulate around the
body, leading to disease.

CHAKRAS
The seven energy points in the body
through which our vital life force passes.
Energy must flow freely through these
points: blocked chakras lead to ill health.

DHATUS
The seven types of tissue that make up
our physical bodies: plasma, blood,
muscle, fat, bone, marrow / nerve, and
reproductive tissue.

DOSHAS
The three energies that make up our mind,
body, and spirit. When the doshas are
balanced, holistic health is maintained, but
any disturbance can lead to illness.

EGO
The part of the mind associated with
conscious thought, the ego is responsible
for our sense of self.

ELEMENTS
There are five elements in the universe
present in everything: ether, air, fire,
water, and earth.

GHEE
Clarified organic butter; used in Ayurveda
in many ways, including for cooking, in
medicines, or on the skin.

HOLISTIC WELLNESS
An approach that considers the whole
person and everything about them, rather
than focusing on individual symptoms.

KAPHA DOSHA
The dosha responsible for structure and
cohesion. Its qualities are heavy, dense,
cold, oily, liquid, slow, smooth, slimy,
static, and sticky.

MALAS
The body's waste products: stools, urine,
and sweat.

MANTRA
A repeated phrase or sound that is used
as part of a healing or meditative practice.

MEDITATION

A practice that usually involves focussing the mind and controlling the breath to help create silence and stillness within, freeing a person from unhelpful thoughts and calming their whole being.

MINDFULNESS

A psychological technique of focusing attention on the here and now, allowing feelings and thoughts to pass without judging or becoming distracted by them, in order to be more in tune with, and aware of, the world around us.

OJAS

The biological substance circulating round our bodies that equates to immunity. It is the end product of all seven tissues being nourished properly. Ojas protects the tissues from the possible damaging effects of imbalanced doshas.

PITTA DOSHA

The dosha responsible for transformation. Its qualities are hot, light, spreading, liquid, sharp, and oily.

PRAKRUTI

A person's *prakruti*, or constitution, is made up of a proportion of the three doshas. This is unique for each individual.

PRANA

The vital life force: describes both the creative energy and power of the universe, and the breath that gives life to every living thing.

SROTAMSI

The channels in our bodies through which substances and vital life force pass.

VATA DOSHA

The dosha responsible for all movement. Its qualities are cold, subtle, rough, clear, dry, mobile, and light.

YOGA

A system of exercises for body and mind; the sister practice of Ayurveda, it helps to unite the mind, body, and spirit.

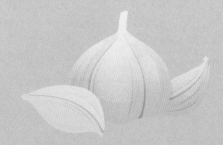

INDEX

Index entries in **bold** indicate specific wellness and healing practices.

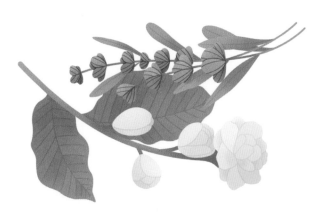

ABOUT THE AUTHOR

Sonja Shah-Williams is the founder and owner of Anala, a private Ayurvedic practice and lifestyle brand in London. She writes regularly about all aspects of holistic health, both for publications and on her website, offering guidance and her own unique modern-day approach to Ayurvedic healing. As well as providing one-on-one consultations and bespoke lifestyle programmes for clients, Sonja also offers training sessions in the basic principles of Ayurveda that can be used to improve all areas of holistic wellbeing. Sonja recently launched her own range of Ayurvedic flower body oils, which she created to bring the ancient Ayurvedic art of anointing to a modern setting.

AUTHOR'S ACKNOWLEDGMENTS

I am eternally grateful to my principal university lecturers, Dr Palitha Serasinghe, Dr Marouf Athique, Dr Venkata Joshi, and Dr Anjali Joshi for their wisdom, humility, and unfailing support during my years of learning. These wonderful souls shone a bright light on the deep layers of Ayurveda that allowed me to absorb its philosophical, scientific, and spiritual significance, and incorporate it into my own psyche. Thank you to my wonderful parents; my late, much missed father, a doctor and visionary, and my darling mother, whose support for everything I do is the embodiment of mother love. Both instilled in me the importance of holistic health and unconditional love.

Thank you to my husband Paul and my children, Jake H and Millie B. Thank you for choosing me to offer you my mother love, which is infinite. Thank you to my brother and sister-in-law, Sunil and Sharmila, Ani my "other daughter" and my sister and brother-in-law, Bella and Del. Thanks to Pat and Ed and the Williams family. Thank you to all members of my Yorkshire Indian family; you know who you are. What a special bond and story we have running through our souls. Thank you to all my amazing girlfriends, for all your love and support. Thank you mostly for being on my life journey with me. Special thanks to the wonderful team at DK: Dawn Henderson, Rona Skene, Louise Brigenshaw, Aimée Longos, Mandy Earey, Kiron Gill, and illustrator Weitong Mai.

PUBLISHER'S ACKNOWLEDGMENTS

DK would like to thank the following for their assistance in the publication of this book: John Friend for proofreading; and Marie Lorimer for compiling the index.